BREAKING THE VICIOUS CIRCLE

THE OLIVER WENDELL HOLMES LECTURES, 1992

The Oliver Wendell Holmes Lectures,
begun in 1941, were established by
the bequest of Oliver Wendell Holmes, Jr.,
Harvard Law School Class of 1866.

BREAKING THE VICIOUS CIRCLE

TOWARD EFFECTIVE RISK REGULATION

STEPHEN BREYER

HARVARD UNIVERSITY PRESS

CAMBRIDGE, MASSACHUSETTS

LONDON, ENGLAND   1993

Library of Congress Cataloging-in-Publication Data
Breyer, Stephen G., 1938–
    Breaking the vicious circle : toward effective risk regulation /
  Stephen Breyer.
      p. cm. — (The Oliver Wendell Holmes Lectures ; 1992)
    Includes bibliographical references and index.
    ISBN 0-674-08114-5 (alk. paper)
    1. Chemicals—Law and legislation—United States.
2. Carcinogens—Safety regulations—United States.   3. Health
risk assessment—United States.   I. Title.   II. Series.
KF3958.B74   1993
353.0082'323—dc20   92-38934
                                                   CIP

To Joanna

CONTENTS

PREFACE

This book is about federal regulation of substances that create health risks. We read almost daily about chemicals that threaten our air, our water, our lives—asbestos, benzene, PCBs, EDB, Agent Orange, Alar, and many others. We hear charges and countercharges: callous industry, greedy lawyers, lives unnecessarily lost, billions of dollars wasted in a pointless search for perfect safety. Were Milton alive, he might describe our present regulatory system as one where "Chaos umpire sits, and by decision more embroils the fray by which he reigns."

How should government deal with such problems? Which substances should we regulate? In what order? To what extent? Who should decide, and how? I shall approach these questions not as a scientist, or an economist, or a regulator, or a member of the public, but as a lawyer interested in the design of governmental institutions. Chapter 1, a substantive analysis, draws on the scientific, technical, and regulatory literature to describe three serious problems with the present regulatory system. Chapter 2, a political analysis, describes possible causes of these problems. Chapter 3, an institutional analysis, draws connections between problems, causes, and potential institutional solutions.

There is a subtext in this book, a subtext that seeks to respond to Oliver Wendell Holmes's admonition to look for the "general" in the "particular." The book suggests a general form of analysis—of underlying substance, political causes, and institutional solutions—that may apply to other public policy problems. I also hope that the book will encourage students of the law to become interested in the general kind of public policy problem I describe, a problem that combines substance, procedure, politics, and administration. Lawyers trying to help create better institutional solutions to important social problems need not simply reason deductively from first principles of procedural fairness or democratic theory. Rather, they can impose those principles as proper constraints, within which they work toward the Platonic goal of every institution—uniting political power with wisdom—so as better to resolve the human problems of our times.

This book, more than most, owes its virtues to the help of many others, who were generous with time, information, and commentary. Let me mention a few of them: members of the Carnegie Commission Task Force on Science and Technology, including its chair, Helene Kaplan, as well as Alvin Alm, Richard Ayres, Douglas Costle, E. Donald Elliott, Richard Merrill, Gil Omenn, Irving Shapiro, and Patricia Wald, and staff members Jonathan Bender, Steven Gallagher, David Robinson, and Mark Schaefer; my colleagues at Harvard, Charles Fried, John Graham, Phil Heymann, and Richard Zeckhauser; scientific and regulatory experts, among them Richard Belzer, Devra Lee Davis, Adam Finkel, Richard Li, Charles Powers, and Richard Stewart; research assistants and helpers, including Kate Adams, Henk Brands, Robert Brauneis, Susan Davies, Jacques deLisle, Simon Frankel, Jeff Lange, Elizabeth Moreno, Aaron Rappaport, Kim Rucker, Simon Steel, and Michael Wynne; and my editor, Michael Aronson.

BREAKING THE
VICIOUS CIRCLE

SYSTEMATIC PROBLEMS | 1

We regulate only some, not all, of the risk that fills the world. Any one of us might be harmed by almost anything—a rotten apple, a broken sidewalk, an untied shoelace, a splash of grapefruit juice, a dishonest lawyer.[1] Regulators try to make our lives safer by eliminating or reducing our exposure to certain potentially risky substances or even persons (unsafe food additives, dangerous chemicals, unqualified doctors). When the regulator focuses upon reducing exposure to a particular substance, when the risk is to health, when the risk is fairly small or uncertain, the regulator typically uses a particular system—a "heartland" regulatory system, the common features of which underlie many different statutory programs.

I focus upon this heartland system, using as an example the regulatory effort to reduce exposure to cancer-causing substances, both because of its illustrative power and because the public's fear of cancer currently drives the system. Still, much of what I say about cancer and similar health risks has broader application to other regulatory screening efforts, for example, whether or not to require seat belts for infants in airplanes, or how to regulate swimming-pool slides.

You need four pieces of background information. First, you need some idea of what I mean by "small risk," the subject of many regulatory programs. The best device I have found for explaining the term is the "risk ladder" prepared by Robert Cameron Mitchell, of Clark University (Figure 1).[2]

About 2.2 million persons die each year in the United States, out of a population of 250 million.[3] Knowing nothing about an individual person, one can assess a crude individual risk of death as just under 1 in 100, or

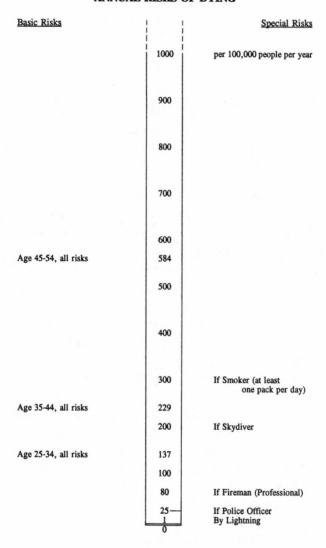

Figure 1. Risk "ladder" showing annual death rates for basic and special risks. *Source:* Robert Cameron Mitchell, Clark University.

LOWER LEVEL RISKS
(Annual)

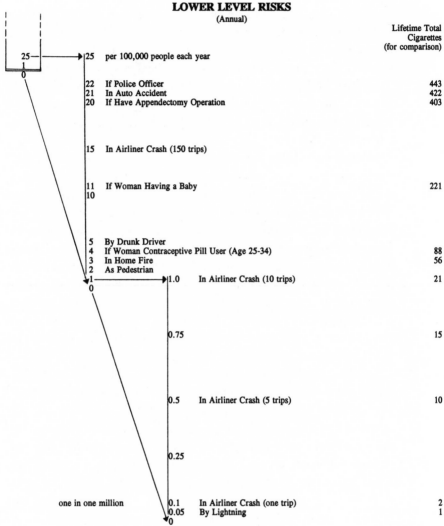

Lifetime Total
Cigarettes
(for comparison)

25	25 per 100,000 people each year	
1		
0		
	22 If Police Officer	443
	21 In Auto Accident	422
	20 If Have Appendectomy Operation	403
	15 In Airliner Crash (150 trips)	
	11 If Woman Having a Baby	221
	10	
	5 By Drunk Driver	
	4 If Woman Contraceptive Pill User (Age 25-34)	88
	3 In Home Fire	56
	2 As Pedestrian	
	1	
	0	
	1.0 In Airliner Crash (10 trips)	21
	0.75	15
	0.5 In Airliner Crash (5 trips)	10
	0.25	
one in one million	0.1 In Airliner Crash (one trip)	2
	0.05 By Lightning	1
	0	

1,000 out of 100,000, as shown at the very top of the figure. If one knows a person's age, one can make a more refined assessment, such as 137 out of 100,000 for all persons between 25 and 34. Certain individuals incur special risks of death because of their professions or their activities. A skydiver, for example, incurs a special annual risk of 200 in 100,000. Those special risks are shown at the right. The enlarged segment of the bottom of the ladder shows special small risks such as the risk of being killed by a drunk driver (5 in 100,000) or being hit by lightning (1 in 2,000,000).

Most people want to ask, "One in a million—is that a lot or a little?" There is no good answer to that question. If one focuses upon statistics, it may seem very little; if one tries to focus upon the 250 or so individual deaths that this number implies (in a population of 250 million), it may seem like a lot. Mitchell, who is an expert in trying to communicate this kind of information neutrally (he employs this chart to help elicit public reactions), uses a "cigarette equivalency" table, shown at the right of the lower-level risk ladder. It indicates that the risk of being hit by lightning is the same as the risk of death from smoking one cigarette once in your life, and it grades other risks accordingly. For present purposes, you should keep in mind that many of the regulatory risks at issue here are in the "blown-up" small-risk portion of the ladder.

Second, you should know a few facts about cancer, the engine that drives much of health risk regulation. Of the 2.2 million Americans who die each year, about 22 percent, or 500,000, die of cancer.[4] Just how many of these deaths are caused by exposure to substances that the government does, or might, regulate (such as chemical pesticides, various pollutants, or food additives) is the subject of considerable scientific dispute. Two leading authorities, Richard Doll and Richard Peto, in the early 1980s published important findings about the causes of cancer deaths (Table 1).[5] The table suggests that pollution and industrial products account for under 3 percent, or less than 15,000, of all cancer deaths, 500,000 per year;[6] other, related scientific work indicates that these and related causes could account for up to 10 percent, or 50,000 deaths. The range of expert estimates seems to be 10,000 to 50,000 deaths, though the more widely accepted view is that only a relatively small portion of these are "regulatable."[7] By way of comparison, consider that smoking-related cancer accounts for 30

Table 1. Proportions of cancer deaths attributed to various factors.

Factor or class of factors	Percent of all cancer deaths	
	Best estimate	Range of acceptable estimates
Tobacco	30	25–40
Alcohol	3	2–4
Diet	35	10–70
Food additives	<1	–5[a]–2
Reproductive and sexual behavior	7	1–13
Occupation	4	2–8
Pollution	2	<1–5
Industrial products	<1	<1–2
Medicines and medical procedures	1	0.5–3
Geophysical factors[b]	3	2–4
Infection	10?	1–?
Unknown	?	?

Source: Richard Doll and Richard Peto, *The Causes of Cancer* 1256 (1981). Reprinted by permission of Oxford University Press.

a. Allowing for a possibly protective effect of antioxidants and other preservatives.

b. Only about 1 percent, not 3 percent, could reasonably be described as "avoidable." Geophysical factors also cause a much greater proportion of nonfatal cancers (up to 30 percent of all cancers, depending on ethnic mix and latitude) because of the importance of UV light in causing the relatively nonfatal basal cell and squamous cell carcinomas of sunlight-exposed skin.

percent, or about 150,000, of those 500,000 deaths.[8] You should also be aware (though this statement is more controversial) that the number of deaths from most of the major types of cancer does not seem to have been increasing, although there is some evidence of increases in the incidence of some, mostly less common, types of cancer.[9] The graph shown in Figure 2, from the American Cancer Society, shows an enormous increase in lung cancer, a decline in stomach and uterine cancers, and a roughly constant incidence of other forms of cancer.[10] In other words, the number of people who die each year from types of cancer whose incidence seems likely to be reduced by regulation is below an estimated ceiling that itself varies between 10,000 and 50,000; it is probably less than 2 percent to 10 percent of all cancer deaths; it is 7 percent to 33 percent of deaths associated with smoking.

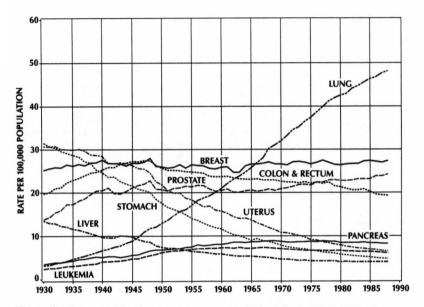

Figure 2. Cancer death rates by site of cancer, United States, 1930–1988. Rates are adjusted to the age distribution of the 1970 census population. Rates are for both sexes combined, except breast and uterine cancer (female population only) and prostate cancer (male population only). *Source:* American Cancer Society, Inc., *Cancer Facts and Figures, 1992.* Used by permission.

The numbers must range from less than 1 percent to less than about 3 percent of our 2.2 million annual mortality total (with the current majority of scientific views closer to the lower end of the spectrum).

Third, you must keep in mind that regulation designed to screen out risky substances, including cancer-causing substances, is embodied in many different regulatory programs—indeed, in at least twenty-six different statutes administered by at least eight different agencies.[11] This alphabet soup of agencies and programs includes such old friends as EPA, DOL, HHS, and NRC, administering, for example, CERCLA,[12] TSCA,[13] FIFRA,[14] CAA,[15] OSHA,[16] FDCA,[17] and AEA.[18] The rules and orders may vary from program to program, sometimes denying permission to market a product, sometimes insisting upon a cleanup, often setting some kind of "dilution" standard above which a product's maker, shipper, or user must provide special handling conditions. Regardless of the precise procedures and rules, however, each agency examines a substance, assesses its health or safety risks, and tries to reduce human contacts that are unacceptably risky.

Fourth, you must have some idea of how the regulatory system works. The system has two basic parts, a technical part, called "risk assessment," designed to measure the risk associated with the substance, and a more policy-oriented part, called "risk management," which decides what to do about it.[19]

Risk assessment can itself be divided into four activities:[20] (a) *Identifying the potential hazard,* say, benzene in respect to cancer: Is it benzene in any context, or just benzene used in industry, or undiluted benzene, or certain solutions of benzene in certain places? (b) *Drawing a dose/response curve:* How does the risk of harm vary with the person's exposure to that substance? The question is critically important, for, as Paracelsus pointed out over four hundred years ago, "the dose alone determines the poison."[21] Drinking a bottle of pure iodine is deadly; placing a drop of diluted iodine on a cut is helpful. Regulators will try to use statistical studies of, say, cancer in humans (epidemiological studies), or experiments with high substance-doses given to animals, to estimate the potential effects of human exposure to low substance-doses over varying periods of time. (c) *Estimating the amount of human exposure:* How many persons in a particular workforce, or in a particular region, or in the public generally, will be exposed to different doses of the substance, and for how long? Suppose exposure to a solution of five parts per million every day for twenty years will be likely to cause five extra deaths per year per million persons. Exposing the entire population may mean 1,250 extra deaths; exposing a hundred thousand persons may mean one extra death every two years. And even in the latter case, if only two persons are exposed to the substance, so that each runs a 50 percent risk of death, there may be a regulatory problem. (d) *Categorizing the result:* Is the substance, in fact, a carcinogen? A strong carcinogen or a weak carcinogen? Based upon the dose/response and exposure findings, how should the risk assessment describe (or categorize) the hazard? In carrying out these activities, particularly in making dose/response and exposure estimates, regulators often find that they simply lack critically important scientific or empirical data: they do not know how many Americans inhale how much benzene at gasoline stations; they do not know the extent to which the biology of a rat or mouse resembles, or differs from, that of a human being. In such instances, they will often make a "default assumption"—a formalized guess—designed to fill the gap and to permit the regulator to continue the analysis.

Risk management determines what the regulator should do about the risks that the assessment reveals. Ideally, the risk manager will consider what will be likely in fact to occur should he choose each of several regulatory options. On the one hand, to what extent will the regulation actually diminish the specific risk at issue? On the other hand, to what extent will regulation itself produce *different* risks? (Will childproof aspirin bottle tops save children, or will they lead many parents, unable to open the top easily, simply to leave the top off?[22] Will saccharin users, denied saccharin, switch to sugar, gain weight, and die of heart attacks?) To what extent will the regulation deprive users of benefits the substance now brings? To what extent will it impose added costs? The manager also must consider practical problems, such as the difficulty of enforcing a regulation or the political reaction that its promulgation might bring. Ultimately, in light of the identified risks, the risks associated with alternatives, the effect on benefits, the costs, and the practicalities, the risk managing regulator will reach a decision.

To summarize: Keep in mind the risk ladder, the 2.2 million annual deaths, the 500,000 annual cancer deaths, the maximum range of 10–50 thousand or so relevant cancer deaths, and the regulatory process aimed at reducing them, a process that involves a risk assessment and a risk management decision.

Major Problems

Three serious problems currently plague efforts to regulate small, but significant, risks to our health. I call these problems *tunnel vision* (or "the last 10 percent"), *random agenda selection,* and *inconsistency.* Scientific, technical, and legal articles in this area confirm that these problems are significant. The literature reveals enormous scientific and technical controversies about facts and predictions related to the regulation of many individual substances (e.g., asbestos, benzene, PCBs, dioxin); it provides good reason for taking many definitive-sounding numerical estimates with a grain (if not a barrel) of salt; yet, at the same time, one can discern a degree of consensus (among many, but never all, reputable experts) about the factual bounds of problems, about orders of magnitude, about limits on the nature of the disagreements. An amateur sailor who cannot locate or describe precisely all the shoals and reefs in a given area may nonetheless determine approximately the size and location of the deep-water channel. Similarly, a judge might provide an impressionistic "report from the literature," rather as he might review a factually techni-cal record, or as a lawyer might assess and report about factual matters relevant to the technically based problems of a client.

You should realize at the outset that, though I believe these three problems are serious enough to warrant institutional change, they do *not* show that EPA, or the other regulatory agencies, are somehow "out of control," or that their staffs are wicked or foolish. To the contrary, EPA generally receives high marks for its work, and the EPA-related problems I describe are but one small aspect of its efforts; my point is to illustrate how well-meaning, intelligent regulators, trying to carry out their regu-latory tasks sensibly, can nonetheless bring about counterproductive results. That is why institutional design is important.

PROBLEM ONE: TUNNEL VISION, OR "THE LAST 10 PERCENT"
Tunnel vision, a classic administrative disease, arises when an agency so organizes or subdivides its tasks that each employee's individual consci-entious performance effectively carries single-minded pursuit of a single goal too far, to the point where it brings about more harm than good. In the regulation of health risks, a more appropriate label is "the last 10 percent," or "going the last mile." The regulating agency considers a substance that poses serious risks, at least through long exposure to high doses. It then promulgates standards so stringent—insisting, for exam-ple, upon rigidly strict site cleanup requirements—that the regulatory action ultimately imposes high costs without achieving significant addi-tional safety benefits. A former EPA administrator put the problem suc-cinctly when he noted that about 95 percent of the toxic material could be removed from waste sites in a few months, but years are spent trying to remove the last little bit.[23] Removing that last little bit can involve limited technological choice, high cost, devotion of considerable agency resources,[24] large legal fees,[25] and endless argument.[26]

Let me provide some examples. The first comes from a case in my own court, *United States v. Ottati & Goss,*[27] arising out of a ten-year effort to force cleanup of a toxic waste dump in southern New Hampshire. The site was mostly cleaned up. All but one of the private parties had settled. The remaining private party litigated the cost of cleaning up the last little bit, a cost of about $9.3 million to remove a small amount of highly diluted PCBs and "volatile organic compounds" (benzene and gasoline components) by incinerating the dirt.[28] How much extra safety did this $9.3 million buy? The forty-thousand-page record of this ten-year effort indicated (and all the parties seemed to agree) that, without the extra expenditure, the waste dump was clean enough for children playing on the site to eat small amounts of dirt daily for 70 days each year without significant harm. Burning the soil would have made it clean enough for the children to eat small amounts daily for 245 days per year without significant harm.[29] But there were no dirt-eating children playing in the area, for it was a swamp.[30] Nor were dirt-eating children likely to appear there, for future building seemed unlikely.[31] The parties also agreed that at least half of the volatile organic chemicals would likely evaporate by the year 2000.[32] To spend $9.3 million to protect non-existent dirt-eating children is what I mean by the problem of "the last 10 percent."

Consider a second, more important, example: asbestos. Asbestos generally comes in two varieties, blue (or amphibole) and white (or chrysotile)—which is the kind found almost uniformly in schools and other public buildings.[33] Most experts believe that undamaged white asbestos left in place is virtually harmless. Asbestos removal stirs up and sends into the air white asbestos fibers that would otherwise remain in place, thus threatening removal workers. That is, the risks accompanying leaving white asbestos in place are so small that removal is likely more dangerous than doing nothing.[34]

Archibald Cox supervised an elaborate study of this highly contentious area, which achieved a near consensus among experts that the risk of death from breathing asbestos inside public buildings is no greater than the risk of death from breathing asbestos outside public buildings, say out on the prairie; and the risk in schools is not significantly greater.[35] A 1990 study, published in *Science,* produced numbers roughly consistent with Cox's report (see Table 2).[36] Annual risks of death in schools from asbestos are probably less than one in ten million; removing all asbestos in the nation as a whole might save between one and twenty-five lives per year, putting

Table 2. Estimates of risk from asbestos exposure in schools in comparison to other risks in U.S. society.

Cause	Annual rate (deaths per million)
Asbestos exposure in schools	0.005–0.093
Whooping cough vaccination (1970–1980)	1–6
Aircraft accidents (1979)	6
High school football (1970–1980)	10
Drowning (ages 5–14)	27
Motor vehicle accident, pedestrian (ages 5–14)	32
Home accidents (ages 1–14)	60
Long-term smoking	1200

Source: Mossman, et al., "Asbestos: Scientific Developments and Implications for Public Policy," 247 *Science* 294, 299 (1990) © AAAS.

Note: Data from six published risk estimates in which total deaths (lung cancer and mesotheliomas) attributable to asbestos exposure over a lifetime were estimated per 1 million students exposed to 0.00024 fibers per cubic centimeter air (the mean airborne concentration in schools) for five school years, beginning at age 10. Estimates indicate that the annual rate is 0.005 to 0.0093 deaths per million students for an average life expectancy of 75 years.

aside the lives of removal workers placed at risk.[37] The article's authors in fact believe that removal "in nonoccupational environments" is the riskier course of action: "the asbestos panic in the U.S. must be curtailed, especially because unwarranted and poorly controlled asbestos abatement results in unnecessary risks to young removal workers."[38]

The risk is so small as to be virtually meaningless. But suppose we ignore the higher risks to removal workers, and ask how much the nation, in fact, may spend to try to lower the direct, non-removal risk. The *Science* article cites removal cost estimates ranging from $53 billion to $150 billion.[39] A mid-range $100 billion figure, assuming a mid-range ten lives saved annually for forty years, means an expenditure of $250 million per statistical life saved over forty years. Is this sensible? We can translate the figure into a more intuitively accessible number by recalling that auto accidents kill about fifty thousand people each year. We might then imagine how much we would willingly pay for a slightly safer car, a car that would reduce auto deaths by, say, 5 percent, to 47,500. Would we pay an extra $1,000 for such a car? An extra $5,000 for that added contribution to safety? To spend $100 billion as a nation to save ten lives annually assumes we value safety so much that each of us would pay $48,077 extra for any such new, slightly safer car.[40] Perhaps the cost estimates are exaggerated. Perhaps Americans are more willing to run voluntary, automobile-related risks, than to run involuntary, school-related risks; perhaps they believe death (at an old age) by cancer is worse than death (at a younger age) in an auto accident. So, let us divide the estimates in half, and in half again. We would still find that the slightly safer car cost over $12,000 extra. Compare airbags, which cost $200 to $500 per car and may save 3,000 to 10,000 lives per year.[41] It seems unlikely that the public would pay 24 to 60 times more per car to save far fewer lives.

A recent Fifth Circuit case[42] shows that such costly efforts to remove asbestos are not theoretical. The Circuit reviewed an agency ban[43] of asbestos pipe, which ban, the agency said, would save one statistical life every four years, or three lives total in thirteen years.[44] The agency banned asbestos shingles, which ban has a one-in-three chance of saving one life total;[45] it banned asbestos coating, which ban, it estimated, would save 3.3 lives total;[46] it banned asbestos paper, which ban has a 60 percent chance of saving one life total.[47] The extra cost of these bans is comparatively low—according to the court, about $200 million to $300 million—but all to save a total of 7–8 lives over thirteen years.[48] If we translate lives saved and costs into our 5 percent safer car comparison, the bans assume a public so safety-conscious its members would pay $6,410 extra for each new, slightly safer car. The Fifth Circuit, striking down the ban, pointed out in a footnote that "over the next 13 years, we can expect more than a dozen deaths from ingested *toothpicks*—a death toll more than twice what the EPA predicts will flow from the quarter-billion-dollar bans of asbestos pipe, shingles, and roof coatings."[49]

Consider a third example, benzene. In 1970, the Occupational Safety and Health Act authorized OSHA to set occupational exposure limits for a range of chemicals, including benzene, a common industrial chemical.[50] In 1978 OSHA promulgated a standard prohibiting worker exposure during any eight-hour period to concentrations of benzene that exceeded one part per million.[51] OSHA had evidence that benzene caused leukemia through longer exposure at higher concentrations. It pointed out that no one knew whether or not benzene caused harm at low concentrations; and, in light of the uncertainty, it imposed the lowest concentration level that industry could feasibly manage, one part per million.[52] In 1980 the Supreme Court held that OSHA had not provided an adequate justification for its choice of a standard below ten parts per million, a level at which harm had been demonstrated.[53]

OSHA then began a seven-year effort to gather evidence.[54] That effort produced considerably more "high concentration/long exposure" evidence of the sort OSHA had the first time.[55] In 1978 it had a Turkish study showing that a hospital in Istanbul had diagnosed leukemia in 31 shoe workers (out of a workforce of 28,500) between 1967 and 1975,[56] and an Italian report stating that 12 persons, out of about 5,000 working with benzene, were diagnosed with leukemia between 1960 and 1963.[57] Later, a U.S. federal agency study found 7 leukemia victims out of 748 rubber film industry workers exposed to benzene in the 1940s;[58] a Dow Chemical study found 3 persons with leukemia among 541 chemical workers exposed to benzene between 1940 and 1970,[59] and many other epidemiological and other animal studies showed that benzene in moderate doses will produce tumors.[60] By applying to this data a mathematical model that assumes benzene produces cancer roughly in proportion to the dose,[61] OSHA found evidence that benzene solutions of as little as one part per million caused harm;[62] it estimated that changing the standard from ten parts to one part per million would save about 8 statistical lives per year for 45 years, at an annual cost of $24 million, or about $3 million per life saved (a comparatively reasonable cost).[63] In the meantime, under the Clean Air Act,[64] EPA declared benzene a hazardous air pollutant and spent ten years, using a different methodology, to create emissions standards for various sources.[65] Experts calculate that the EPA rules, regulating sources such as benzene storage vessels and coke by-product recovery plants, save a total of 3 to 4 lives per year, at a cost of well over $200 million; one regulation costs approximately $180 million to save a single statistical life.[66]

The upshot, in OSHA's case, is years of agency time and effort, many studies, and lengthy hearings to obtain mathematically related figures that OSHA (had it guessed what the Supreme Court would say) might have produced the first time. The upshot, in EPA's case, is an expenditure of considerable effort to achieve results that save very few lives at very high cost.

At this point, you may interrupt with a few questions: "Who is to say whether $1 million, or $10 million, or $240 million, or $10 billion, is too much, or too little, to spend to save eight or eighteen or eighty statistical lives? Who can value a human life?"[67]

I cannot answer these questions except by pointing out that, every day, each of us implicitly evaluates risks to life. We begin to run risks to achieve our daily objectives the instant we get out of bed. We find it worth spending money on an ordinary fire alarm system, but not worth installing state-of-the-art automatic-phone-dialing fire protection. We believe it worth installing guard rails on bridges, but not worth coating the Grand Canyon in soft plastic to catch those who might fall over the edge.

"But don't people value different risks differently?" you ask. "Might they not particularly fear cancer, or strongly believe the government should pay to eliminate risks from involuntary exposure, say, to asbestos, rather than risks associated with voluntary activities, such as driving or football?"

The answer is yes. Indeed, psychologists have studies that try to show how people value the same numerical risks differently depending upon such factors. Figure 3, from such a study, shows dots of different sizes, each size representing a higher value placed on avoiding the same numerical risk depending upon the "dread" or the "unknowability" of circumstances with which it is associated.[68] To this extent, auto safety and asbestos safety are dissimilar. But if you think it is reasonable to spend more money to save a life when asbestos is at issue, you must, at least, ask yourself how much more, and you should try to explain to yourself why. It seems to me unlikely that such value differences could explain my examples.

"No regulatory system is perfect," you might add. "Does it really matter if occasionally the nation spends a little too much money buying a little too much safety? After all, every scientific study is filled with uncertainties that the final, specific numbers tend to hide. Why not err on the safe side?"

This question is critically important. My answer has two parts. First, the literature contains too many examples for the reader to conclude that the small-dose problem, overall, is itself small enough to shrug aside. Leaving aside the morality of the Vietnam war, is Agent Orange in fact a dangerous, cancer-causing substance? The federal judge who heard the

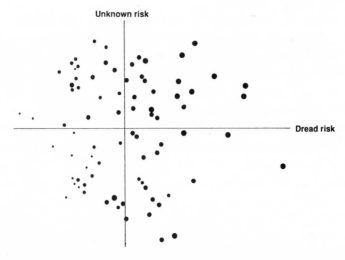

Figure 3. Attitudes toward regulation of hazards. The larger the point, the greater the desire for strict regulation to reduce risk. *Source:* Paul Slovic, "Perception of Risk," 236 *Science* 283 (1987) © AAAS.

case, Jack Weinstein, wrote that the evidence suggested the plaintiffs' case was "without merit" and [69] that a "directed verdict" for defendants "would be required."[70] Many studies support that conclusion.[71]

How dangerous are the fearsome-sounding PCBs? We know that exposure to high concentrations causes rashes in humans and tumors in test animals. But should the EPA have set a standard for transformers leaking PCB-laden mineral oil so low as to require the expenditure of $140 million to avoid health risks considerably lower than those accompanying eating a raw mushroom?[72] How broadly should regulatory agencies have swept with their ban of EDB, a grain fumigant which under most circumstances poses risks roughly equivalent to those posed by the chloroform in chlorine to the child who spends an hour in a swimming pool?[73] A total ban could lead farmers to switch to other, more dangerous fumigants instead, or lead them to fumigate their crops less well, leaving more mold residues, which bring with them an increased cancer risk from aflatoxin.[74] One also reads that one recent hazardous waste land-disposal ban required spending $4 billion to save one statistical life,[75] that one drinking-water standard limited daily risks from polynuclear aromatic hydrocarbons (PAHs) to those typically found in two slices of bread per day (or a ten-ounce steak every two months),[76] that EPA's "uranium mill tailings" standard hoped to save six lives per year as a "plausible upper bound,"[77] that all EPA regulation, working perfectly, would prevent 1200 to 6600 cancer deaths per year,[78] and that about 90 percent of the expenditure by insurers, and about 20 percent of the expenditure by firms held liable, under Superfund has gone for legal fees and other transaction costs, rather than for cleanup.[79] Each of these examples individually has controversial aspects, but taken together they illustrate a significant "last 10 percent" problem.

The second reason that it matters whether the nation spends too much to buy a little extra safety is that the resources available to combat health risks are not limitless.[80] Consider such present-system cost estimates as a *New York Times* survey of experts predicting that total toxic waste cleanup costs will mushroom to $300–700 billion (see Table 3),[81] a university study suggesting various toxic site cleanup costs of $245–700 billion,[82] a Mitre Corporation estimate of total Superfund cleanup costs of as much as $1 trillion,[83] and a Department of Energy estimate of its (quite separate) nuclear site cleanup costs of $240 billion.[84] Compare these numbers with the total of $100–120 billion annually the federal government now spends to protect all aspects of the environment.[85] If we take the $9.3 million spent on the New Hampshire waste dump cleanup[86] as an indicator of the general problem of

Table 3. The cost of cleaning up several categories of polluted sites.

Category	Number of sites (estimated)	Estimated cost ($ billions)
Superfund abandoned sites	4,000	$80–120
Federally owned sites	5,000–10,000	75–250
Corrective action on active private sites	2,000–5,000	12–100
Leaking underground storage tanks	350,000–400,000	32
State law mandated cleanups	6,000–12,000	3–120+
Inactive uranium tailings	24	1.3
Abandoned mine lands	22,300	55

Source: New York Times, September 1, 1991, p. 28. Copyright © 1991 by the New York Times Company. Reprinted by permission.

high costs in trying for that "last 10 percent" ($9.3 million[87] times 26,000 toxic waste dumps[88] is $242 billion), we have an answer to the question, "Does it matter if we spend too much over-insuring our safety?" The money is not, or will not be, there to spend, at least not if we want to address more serious environmental or social problems— the need for better prenatal care, vaccinations,[89] and cancer diagnosis, let alone daycare, housing, and education. For example, one study suggests that vaccinating 18-month-olds against hemophilus influenza Type b, the leading cause of bacterial meningitis, would save toddlers' lives at the comparatively tiny cost of $68,000 each.[90] Similarly, a large-scale study conducted in the Netherlands found that a far-reaching mammography program would save thousands of lives at a cost of about $54,000 each.[91] While several states have instituted limited screening programs for breast cancer, there is no national effort to encourage and fund regular examinations.

In sum, the "dirt-eating children" example offers a powerful argument, as we shall see later, not necessarily for deregulation, but for a serious effort to prioritize, and perhaps to reallocate, our regulatory resources.

PROBLEM TWO: RANDOM AGENDA SELECTION

The literature also suggests a serious problem with the creation of regulatory agendas and with the establishment of rational priorities among the items that are included in those agendas. Since regulators will normally act against a major risk that comes to the public's attention, it is more difficult than with the first problem to find examples, for they must be examples of what is *not* being done.

Some critics point out that, of the more than sixty thousand chemical substances potentially subject to regulation,[92] only a few thousand have undergone more than crude toxicity testing.[93] The General Accounting Office, for example, after a recent examination of EPA's testing agenda, under the 1976 Toxic Substances Control Act, found that the relevant EPA Committee had recommended only 386 substances for testing as of 1990.[94] The GAO wrote that the testing program "has made little progress,"[95] that EPA "has received complete test data for only six chemicals,"[96] that the untested chemicals, in all likelihood, include harmful chemicals,[97] and that the agency has no particular strategy for determining which of these many chemicals are likely to need testing and which are not.[98] Of course, serious carcinogenic testing is expensive, costing perhaps more than $1 million per chemical.[99] But the critics complain of not enough effort to create a systematic testing procedure better able to identify the more serious risks first.[100]

Other critics complain of a regulatory overemphasis on cancer risks, compared with other, possibly greater risks, such as the risk of neurotoxicity, causing potential brain damage.[101] Several years ago, for example, the National Institute for Occupational Health and Safety estimated that nearly ten million workers are exposed daily, through inhalation or skin contact, to solvents.[102] All solvents produce some adverse nervous-system effects at some level. While some neurotoxins are regulated as carcinogens, neurotoxic effects receive little special attention.[103]

Most significant, in my view, is the EPA's own, now famous, 1987 report called "Unfinished Business." In that report EPA managers provided their own views of proper program priority rankings and compared them with existing priorities. Subjects that risk managers ranked low, such as hazardous waste cleanup, had high funding priorities; subjects that they ranked high, such as indoor air pollution and global warming, had low funding priorities.[104] In 1990 EPA's Science Advisory Board conducted a similar exercise and, after careful study, confirmed the risk managers' views.[105] The general public's ranking of safety priorities is very different from these experts' views (see Table 4).[106] Agency priorities and agendas may more closely reflect public rankings, politics, history, or even chance than the kind of priority list that environmental experts would deliberately create. To a degree, that is inevitable. But one cannot find any detailed federal governmental list that prioritizes health or safety risk problems so as to create a rational, overall agenda—an agenda that would seek to maximize attainable safety or to minimize health-related harms.

If you go to the Air and Space Museum in Washington, D.C., and look at satellite photos of Madagascar, you see a landscape no longer green with trees, but entirely red as its rivers carry the uncovered soil's clay to the sea. To consider the climate-warming health-related consequences of this process, while thinking of our efforts to protect New Hampshire's nonexistent dirt-eating children, helps to underscore the need for rational, problem-related agendas.

Table 4. How the public and EPA rate health risks associated with
environmental problems.

Public	EPA experts
1. Hazardous waste sites	Medium-to-low
2. Exposure to worksite chemicals	High
3. Industrial pollution of waterways	Low
4. Nuclear accident radiation	Not ranked
5. Radioactive waste	Not ranked
6. Chemical leaks from underground storage tanks	Medium-to-low
7. Pesticides	High
8. Pollution from industrial accidents	Medium-to-low
9. Water pollution from farm runoff	Medium
10. Tap water contamination	High
11. Industrial air pollution	High
12. Ozone layer destruction	High
13. Coastal water contamination	Low
14. Sewage-plant water pollution	Medium-to-low
15. Vehicle exhaust	High
16. Oil spills	Medium-to-low
17. Acid rain	High
18. Water pollution from urban runoff	Medium
19. Damaged wetlands	Low
20. Genetic alteration	Low
21. Non-hazardous waste sites	Medium-to-low
22. Greenhouse effect	Low
23. Indoor air pollution	High
24. X-ray radiation	Not ranked
25. Indoor radon	High
26. Microwave oven radiation	Not ranked

Source: Frederick Allen, U.S. EPA, based on EPA report "Unfinished Business: A
Comparative Assessment of Environmental Problems" (1987) and national public opinion
polls by the Roper Organization in December 1987 and January 1988.

PROBLEM THREE: INCONSISTENCY

A final problem that the literature suggests is serious inconsistencies
within and among both programs and agencies. First, agencies use different methods for estimating the effects of their regulations. Thus, a
Resources for the Future expert, trying to estimate the number of cancer
deaths EPA regulations might prevent, was forced to estimate about
6,400 lives saved using EPA's methods of calculation, but only about
1,400 using FDA's methods—a five-fold discrepancy.[107]

Second, irrespective of different calculation methods, the values that regulators implicitly attach to the saving of a statistical life vary widely from one program or agency to another. OMB's 1992 study shows variations ranging from space heater regulations that save lives at a cost of $100,000 per life saved to bans on DES in cattle feed that require an expenditure of $125 million per statistical life (Table 5).[108] (OMB calculated that one minor regulation cost $5.7 trillion per life saved, which calculation probably means only that OMB thought it saved no one.)[109] By way of comparison, statistical studies indicate that labor unions, when free to bargain about safety rules, will insist upon rules that value statistical lives saved at around $5–6 million.[110] These estimates suggest that the nation could buy more safety by refocusing its regulatory efforts.

Third, one can find many examples of regulators' ignoring one program's safety or environmental effects upon another, which suggests a need for interprogram coordination. Proposed rules concerning disposal of sewage sludge, designed to save one statistical life every five years, would encourage waste incineration likely to cause two statistical cancer deaths annually.[111] Rules designed to limit zinc in water raise the cost of using regular diapers, encouraging the use of disposable—and doubtfully "recyclable"—diapers, which are a major contributor to landfills.[112] At one time, EPA's Office of Solid Waste and Emergency Response had designated trace levels of carbon tetrachloride and chloroform found in chlorofluorocarbons (CFCs) as hazardous waste, thus severely discouraging (with the threat of Superfund liability) the recycling of refrigerators, which contain CFCs, while EPA's Office of Air and Radiation was urging that refrigerators be recycled to save the ozone layer. The FDA, meanwhile, was—and remains—content with the use of the same CFCs in asthma inhalers.[113] In 1989 the National Highway Traffic Safety Authority refused to make automobile fuel consumption standards less stringent, despite evidence that, by encouraging manufacturers to market smaller, less crash-resistant cars, the stringency of the regulations may have been costing hundreds of lives per year. According to Judge Stephen Williams, the NHTSA failed to address the lives-for-fuel tradeoff, instead "cowering behind bureaucratic mumbo-jumbo."[114] Again, despite the controversies surrounding each individual example here cited,[115] the instances are sufficient in number to produce an overall impression of an interprogram, interagency coordination problem.

Fourth, and perhaps most seriously, the regulation of small risks can produce inconsistent results, for it can cause more harm to health than it prevents. Sometimes risk estimates leave out important countervailing lethal effects, such as the effect of floating asbestos fibers on passersby or on asbestos-removal workers (who, in fact, do not wear completely protective clothing).[116] Sometimes the regulator does not, or cannot easily, take account of offsetting consumer behavior, as, for example, when a farmer, deprived of his small-cancer-risk artificial pesticide, grows a new, hardier crop variety that contains more "natural pesticides" which may be equally or more carcinogenic (99.99 percent of all pesticides in food, measured by weight, are "natural," according to one scientist, Bruce Ames).[117]

At all times regulation imposes costs that mean less real income available to individuals for alternative expenditure. That deprivation of real income itself has adverse health effects, in the form of poorer diet, more heart attacks, more suicides.[118] To obtain an order of magnitude, a sample of academic studies suggests, as a conservative estimate, that every $7.25 million spent on a cleanup regulation will, under certain assumptions, induce one additional fatality through this "income effect";[119] that a 1 percent increase in unemployment, sustained over five years, means 19,000 more heart attacks and 1,100 more suicides over that time;[120] and that risk varies inversely with family income such that "a 1 percent change in income reduces mortality by about 0.05 percent on average."[121] One need not take these studies as quantitatively accurate. They show only small negative income effects. Where regulation aims at large risks, this small counterproductive tendency is irrelevant; where regulation aims at tiny risks, however, these small negative offsetting consequences mean that a costly standard that seeks to save a few statistical lives more likely saves no lives at all, on balance.[122]

Finally, the literature suggests many concrete possibilities for obtaining increased health, safety, and environmental benefits through reallocation of regulatory resources.[123] Consider the following possible courses: advertising the cancer-causing potential of sunbathing, indoor smoke and pollution, and radon[124] and subsidizing the creation of healthier indoor climates;[125] encouraging changes in diet to avoid natural carcinogens;[126] encouraging or requiring manufacturers to conduct "environmental audits";[127] financing investigations of cancer-causing diets

Table 5. Risks and Cost-Effectiveness of Selected Regulations (from the Budget for Fiscal Year 1992, Table C-2, Part 2, p. 370).

Regulation[a]	Year issued
Unvented Space Heater Ban	1980
Aircraft Cabin Fire Protection Standard	1985
Auto Passive Restraint/Seat Belt Standards	1984
Steering Column Protection Standard[b]	1967
Underground Construction Standards[c]	1989
Trihalomethane Drinking Water Standards	1979
Aircraft Seat Cushion Flammability Standard	1984
Alcohol and Drug Control Standards[c]	1985
Auto Fuel-System Integrity Standard	1975
Standards for Servicing Auto Wheel Rims[c]	1984
Aircraft Floor Emergency Lighting Standard	1984
Concrete & Masonry Construction Standards[c]	1988
Crane Suspended Personnel Platform Standard	1988
Passive Restraints for Trucks & Buses (Proposed)	1989
Side-Impact Standards for Autos (Dynamic)	1990
Children's Sleepwear Flammability Ban[d]	1973
Auto Side Door Support Standards	1970
Low-Altitude Windshear Equipment & Training Standards	1988
Electrical Equipment Standards (Metal Mines)	1970
Trenching and Excavation Standards[c]	1989
Traffic Alert and Collision Avoidance (TCAS) Systems	1988
Hazard Communication Standard[c]	1983
Side-Impact Standards for Trucks, Buses, and MPVs (Proposed)	1989
Grain Dust Explosion Prevention Standards[c]	1987
Rear Lap/Shoulder Belts for Autos	1989
Standards for Radionuclides in Uranium Mines[c]	1984
Benzene NESHAP (Original: Fugitive Emissions)	1984
Ethylene Dibromide Drinking Water Standard	1991
Benzene NESHAP (Revised: Coke Byproducts)[c]	1988
Asbestos Occupational Exposure Limit[c]	1972
Benzene Occupational Exposure Limit[c]	1987

Health or safety	Agency	Baseline mortality risk per million exposed	Cost per premature death averted ($millions 1990)
S	CPSC	1,890	0.1
S	FAA	5	0.1
S	NHTSA	6,370	0.1
S	NHTSA	385	0.1
S	OSHA-S	38,700	0.1
H	EPA	420	0.2
S	FAA	11	0.4
H	FRA	81	0.4
S	NHTSA	343	0.4
S	OSHA-S	630	0.4
S	FAA	2	0.6
S	OSHA-S	630	0.6
S	OSHA-S	81,000	0.7
S	NHTSA	6,370	0.7
S	NHTSA	NA	0.8
S	CPSC	29	0.8
S	NHTSA	2,520	0.8
S	FAA	NA	1.3
S	MSHA	NA	1.4
S	OSHA-S	14,310	1.5
S	FAA	NA	1.5
S	OSHA-S	1,800	1.6
S	NHTSA	NA	2.2
S	OSHA-S	9,450	2.8
S	NHTSA	NA	3.2
H	EPA	6,300	3.4
H	EPA	1,470	3.4
H	EPA	NA	5.7
H	EPA	NA	6.1
H	OSHA-H	3,015	8.3
H	OSHA-H	39,600	8.9

Table 5 (continued)

Regulation[a]	Year issued
Electrical Equipment Standards (Coal Mines)[c]	1970
Arsenic Emission Standards for Glass Plants	1986
Ethylene Oxide Occupational Exposure Limit[c]	1984
Arsenic/Copper NESHAP	1986
Hazardous Waste Listing for Petroleum Refining Sludge	1990
Cover/Move Uranium Mill Tailings (Inactive Sites)	1983
Benzene NESHAP (Revised: Transfer Operations)	1990
Cover/Move Uranium Mill Tailings (Active Sites)	1983
Acrylonitrile Occupational Exposure Limit[c]	1978
Coke Ovens Occupational Exposure Limit[c]	1976
Lockout/Tagout[c]	1989
Asbestos Occupational Exposure Limit[c]	1986
Arsenic Occupational Exposure Limit[c]	1978
Asbestos Ban	1989
Diethylstilbestrol (DES) Cattlefeed Ban	1979
Benzene NESHAP (Revised: Waste Operations)	1990
1,2-Dichloropropane Drinking Water Standard	1991
Hazardous Waste Land Disposal Ban (1st 3rd)	1988
Municipal Solid Waste Landfill Standards (Proposed)	1988
Formaldehyde Occupational Exposure Limit[c]	1987
Atrazine/Alachlor Drinking Water Standard	1991
Hazardous Waste Listing for Wood-Preserving Chemicals	1990

Source: Regulatory Program of the United States Government, April 1, 1991–March 31, 1992, p. 12.

a. 70-year lifetime exposure assumed unless otherwise specified.
b. 50-year lifetime exposure.
c. 45-year lifetime exposure.
d. 12-year exposure period.
NA—not available.

Agency abbreviations: CPSC: Consumer Product Safety Commission; MSHA: Mine Safety and Health Administration; EPA: Environmental Protection Agency; NHTSA: National Highway Traffic Safety Administration; FAA: Federal Aviation Administration; FRA: Federal Railroad Administration; FDA: Food and Drug Administration; OSHA-H: Occupational Safety and Health Administration, Health Standards; OSHA-S: Occupational Safety and Health Administration, Safety Standards.

Health or safety	Agency	Baseline mortality risk per million exposed	Cost per premature death averted ($millions 1990)
S	MSHA	NA	9.2
H	EPA	2,660	13.5
H	OSHA-H	1,980	20.5
H	EPA	63,000	23.0
H	EPA	210	27.6
H	EPA	30,100	31.7
H	EPA	NA	32.9
H	EPA	30,100	45.0
H	OSHA-H	42,300	51.5
H	OSHA-H	7,200	63.5
S	OSHA-S	4	70.9
H	OSHA-H	3,015	74.0
H	OSHA-H	14,800	106.9
H	EPA	NA	110.7
H	FDA	22	124.8
H	EPA	NA	168.2
H	EPA	NA	653.0
H	EPA	2	4,190.4
H	EPA	<1	19,107.0
H	OSHA-H	31	86,201.8
H	EPA	NA	92,069.7
H	EPA	<1	5,700,000.0

and subsidizing the production of healthier foods; paying for early cancer screenings and patients' travel to central cancer hospitals; subsidizing the purchase or installation of smoke detectors; spending more governmental time and effort on more serious ecological problems, such as ozone, forest destruction, or climate change; and raising funds for some of the above by taxing low-risk carcinogens. Such alternatives are closely related to health. But they do not now readily find their way onto the agendas of regulators who must act chemical by chemical or substance by substance.

The upshot is inconsistency that suggests something even more serious than a need for reallocation. When we treat tiny, moderate, and large risks too much alike, we begin to resemble the boy who cried "wolf." Who now reads the warnings on aspirin bottles, or the pharmaceutical drug warnings that run on, in tiny print, for several pages? Will a public that hears these warnings too often and too loudly begin too often to ignore them?[128] Will there be a public reaction that fails to take account of serious risks?

Two years ago, while jogging near the Charles River, I noticed that the footpath was closed to prevent joggers from going through a tunnel where workers had earlier been removing asbestos. Because of bad planning, the path leading to the tunnel's mouth remained open. Rather than go back a half mile to another path, most joggers just dashed madly across Storrow Drive, dodging traffic, and continued on their way. That morning jog might stand as a symbol for Problem Three.

In considering my examples, you must remember several important caveats. These examples are selective; they focus on extremes. They leave out the far more numerous examples of balanced, sensible, and cost-effective regulations. The examples are meant to suggest, though they do not prove, that the smaller the risks at issue, the more likely the costs will be excessive. A larger view of the broader regulatory landscape would reveal, in respect to moderate or large risks, far less problematic results. My examples omit many qualifications; you must recall that the subject is filled with technical uncertainty and disagreement. The examples also are suggestive, not determinative: I cannot *prove* that efforts to achieve "the last 10 percent" will cost billions of dollars; I can simply provide rough estimates of magnitudes for total program costs, along with reasons for thinking that pursuing "the last 10 percent" poses a serious problem.

Still, by means of my examples, I believe one can discover a fairly widespread view, within a knowledgeable community, that efforts to regulate small risks to health are plagued by serious problems of tunnel vision, random agenda selection, and inconsistency.

CAUSES: THE VICIOUS CIRCLE | 2

I n considering the causes of the regulatory problems identified in
Chapter 1, I wish to consider how public perceptions, Congressional
actions and reactions, and technical regulatory methods reinforce
each other. They tend to create a vicious circle, diminishing public trust
in regulatory institutions and thereby inhibiting more rational regulation.
Congress reacts to the public and influences the regulators, who, in their
choice of methods and problems, in turn influence both public perception
and Congressional reaction. Understanding the interaction of these three
elements will suggest what we can and cannot change.

Public Perceptions

Study after study shows that the public's evaluation of risk problems
differs radically from any consensus of experts in the field.[1] Risks
associated with toxic waste dumps and nuclear power appear near the
bottom of most expert lists; they appear near the top of the public's
list of concerns, which more directly influences regulatory agendas (see
Table 4 and Table 6). To some extent, these differences may reflect that
the public fears certain risks more than others with the same probability
of harm. As previously pointed out, of two equal risks, one could rationally
dislike or fear more the risk that is involuntarily suffered, new, unobserv-
able, uncontrollable, catastrophic, delayed, a threat to future generations,
or likely accompanied by pain or dread.[2]

Still, these differences in the source, quality, or nature of a risk may
not account for the different ranking by the public and the experts. A
typical member of the public would like to minimize risks of death to

Table 6. Ordering of perceived risk for thirty activities and technologies.

Activity or technology	League of Women Voters	College students	Active club members	Experts
Nuclear power	1	1	8	20
Motor vehicles	2	5	3	1
Handguns	3	2	1	4
Smoking	4	3	4	2
Motorcycles	5	6	2	6
Alcoholic beverages	6	7	5	3
General (private) aviation	7	15	11	12
Police work	8	8	7	17
Pesticides	9	4	15	8
Surgery	10	11	9	5
Firefighting	11	10	6	18
Large construction	12	14	13	13
Hunting	13	18	10	23
Spray cans	14	13	23	26
Mountain climbing	15	22	12	29
Bicycles	16	24	14	15
Commercial aviation	17	16	18	16
Electric power (non-nuclear)	18	19	19	9
Swimming	19	30	17	10
Contraceptives	20	9	22	11
Skiing	21	25	16	30
X-rays	22	17	24	7
High school and college football	23	26	21	27
Railroads	24	23	29	19
Food preservatives	25	12	28	14
Food coloring	26	20	30	21
Power mowers	27	28	25	28
Prescription antibiotics	28	21	26	24
Home appliances	29	27	27	22
Vaccinations	30	29	29	25

Source: Paul Slovic, "Perception of Risk," 236 Science 280, 281 (1987) © AAAS.

Note: Ordering is based on the geometric mean risk ratings within each group. Rank 1 represents the most risky activity or technology.

himself, to his family, to his neighbors; he would normally prefer that regulation buy more safety for a given expenditure or the same amount of safety for less. Not many of us would like to shift resources to increase overall risks of death significantly in order to increase the likelihood that death will occur on a bicycle or in a fire, rather than through disease. There is a far simpler explanation for the public's aversion to toxic waste dumps than an enormous desire for supersafety, or a strong aversion to the tiniest risk of harm—namely, the public does not *believe* that the risks are tiny. The public's "nonexpert" reactions reflect not different values but different understandings about the underlying risk-related facts.[3]

My assumption that the public assigns "rational" values to risks, however, does not entail rational public reactions to risk. Psychologists have found several examples of thinking that impede rational understanding, but may have helped us survive as we lived throughout much of prehistory, in small groups of hunter-gatherers, depending upon grain, honey, and animals for sustenance. The following, rather well-documented aspects of risk perception are probably familiar.[4]

1. *Rules of thumb.* In daily life most of us do not weigh all the pros and cons of feasible alternatives. We use rules of thumb, more formally called "heuristic devices."[5] We simplify radically; we reason with the help of a few readily understandable examples; we categorize (events and other people) in simple ways that tend to create binary choices—yes/no, friend/foe, eat/abstain, safe/dangerous, act/don't act—and may reflect deeply rooted aversions, such as fear of poisons.[6] The resulting categorizations do not always accurately describe another person or circumstance, but they help us make quick decisions, most of which prove helpful.[7] This kind of quick decision-making may help cut a swath through the modern information jungle, but it oversimplifies dramatically and thereby inhibits an understanding of risks, particularly small risks.[8]

2. *Prominence.* People react more strongly, and give greater importance, to events that stand out from the background. Unusual events are striking.[9] We more likely notice the (low-risk) nuclear waste disposal truck driving past the school than the (much higher-risk) gasoline delivery trucks on their way to local service stations. Journalists, whose job is to write interesting stories, know this psychological fact well.[10] The American Medical Association examined how the press treated two similar stories, one finding increased leukemia rates among nuclear

workers, the other finding no increased cancer rates among those living near nuclear plants. More than half of the newspapers in the study mentioned the first story but not the second; and more than half of those that mentioned both emphasized the first.[11]

3. *Ethics.* The strength of our feelings of ethical obligation seems to diminish with distance. That is to say, feelings of obligation are stronger (or we have different, more time-consuming obligations) toward family, neighbors, friends, community, and those with whom we have direct contact, those whom we see, than toward those who live in distant places, whom we do not see but only read or hear about.

4. *Trust in experts.* People cannot easily judge between experts when those experts disagree with each other. The public, since the mid-1960s, has shown increasing distrust of experts and the institutions, private, academic, or governmental, that employ them.[12]

5. *Fixed decisions.* A person who has made up his or her mind about something is very reluctant to change it.

6. *Mathematics.* Most people have considerable difficulty understanding the mathematical probabilities involved in assessing risk (see Table 7). People consistently overestimate small probabilities. What is the likelihood of death by botulism? (One in two million.) They underestimate large ones. What is the likelihood of death by diabetes? (One in fifty thousand.)[13] People cannot detect inconsistencies in their own risk-related choices. Ask a friend two questions: (1) "Which escape route, Path A or Path B, should the general take with his six hundred soldiers? Path A means two hundred soldiers are saved for certain; Path B means a two-thirds chance that all die, a one-third chance that all are saved." Most people prefer A. (2) "Which escape route, Path A or Path B, should the general take with his six hundred soldiers? Path A means four hundred soldiers die for certain; Path B means a one-third chance that all are saved and a two-thirds chance that all will die." Most people prefer B. They do not realize that the two questions are the same and that their answers are inconsistent. The words "saved" and "die" make the difference. The way one phrases a question can determine people's preferences.[14] Moreover, people do not understand the counterintuitive consequence of certain important statistical propositions. Consider the statistical fact that after any unusually high or low result, the next instance will tend to "deviate toward the mean," which is why parents

Table 7. The frequency of dramatic and sensational lethal events tends to be overestimated; the frequency of unspectacular events tends to be underestimated.

Most overestimated	Most underestimated
All accidents	Smallpox vaccination
Motor vehicle accidents	Diabetes
Pregnancy, childbirth, and abortion	Stomach cancer
Tornadoes	Lightning
Flood	Stroke
Botulism	Tuberculosis
All cancer	Asthma
Fire and flames	Emphysema
Venomous bite or sting	
Homicide	

Source: Baruch Fischhoff, "Managing Risk Perceptions," *Issues in Science and Technology,* vol. 2, no. 1 (Fall 1985). Copyright 1985 by the National Academy of Sciences, Washington, D.C. Reprinted by permission.

who are particularly intelligent, or particularly stupid, tend to have more normal children. Now imagine a teacher who rewards a student's unusually good performance; the next time the student will likely do worse (just because of deviation toward the mean). The same teacher punishes an unusually bad performance; the next time the student will likely do better (just because of the law of averages). The teacher, seeing these results, thinks there is something wrong with the teaching theory of "positive reinforcement." There isn't. Instead, the statistical deviation toward the mean is positively reinforcing the teacher's negative reinforcement, and negatively reinforcing the positive reinforcement.[15] Now, do you understand why students sometimes complain about the harshness of law school professors?

These few, near-commonsense propositions, with strong statistical support in the technical literature, verify Oliver Wendell Holmes's own observation that "most people think dramatically, not quantitatively."[16] They also have important consequences. Consider the public reaction to toxic waste dumps. Start with the mathematical facts about the probability of various occurrences: In 1985 a New Jersey woman won the state lottery twice.[17] What are the odds against this, billions to one? Given the vast number of lotteries in the world, the odds come close to favoring someone somewhere winning a lottery twice. Given the population of the world, and the number of dreams each night, the odds favor someone somewhere dreaming he marries a girl who looks very much like the girl he meets the next day and marries. Given the number of toxic waste dumps in the United States (26,000) and the number of places with above-average cancer rates (half of all places), obviously many cities, towns, and rural areas near toxic waste dumps must also have seriously elevated cancer rates ("mathematics").

Add what sells newspapers—interesting stories—and you can be fairly certain the press will write about the double lottery-winner, perhaps the dreamer, and, if the mathematical evidence is somewhat less crude than my example, the toxic waste dump ("prominence"). Will it be easy to convince the cancer victim that the waste dump (water that is "pure" or "not pure") had nothing to do with the disease ("rules of thumb")? And how will the public react to the image of the angry family member on nightly television ("ethics"), particularly if experts disagree ("trust in experts")—as they might, for the relation between the disease and the toxic site may not be strictly chance (the lottery, too, might be fixed). If further study exonerates the dump, will the viewing public change its mind ("fixed decision")?[18]

When we think about nuclear power controversies, we should take account of the fact that hearing about an accident is what psychologists tell us is an heuristic "tip-off" of danger, whether or not anyone is hurt.[19] We have "seen" Chernobyl and Three Mile Island, and we may therefore doubt nuclear power's safety, whether or not experts tell us that the reactor at Chernobyl was not properly designed, that the accident at Three Mile Island hurt no one, that military weapons, not electric power generators, are responsible for 99 percent of all nuclear waste, that nuclear power's risks are minuscule compared to the risks of coal-generated power. Add a few disagreements among experts and the fact that most members of the public made up their minds long ago, and one can understand nuclear power's position on the public perception risk charts.

These few propositions suggest that better "risk communications," such as efforts to explain risks to the public at open meetings, may not suffice to alleviate risk regulation problems. It is not surprising that, after the EPA Administrator William Ruckelshaus spent days at such meetings in Tacoma, Washington, explaining why an ASARCO chemical plant that was leaking small amounts of arsenic could remain open, he was misunderstood, criticized, and accused of trying to drive a wedge between environmentalists and blue collar workers. The plant eventually closed, although perhaps for other reasons.[20] Nor is it surprising that after special public discussions of nuclear power plants were held in Sweden, surveys of the eighty thousand Swedes who participated showed no consensus, but increased confusion.[21]

There is little reason to hope for better risk communication over time. To the contrary, as science improves, scientists may more easily detect and identify ever tinier risks—the risks associated, for example, with the migration of a single molecule of plastic from a container into a soft drink; they may more easily identify geographical areas near toxic waste dumps with higher than average cancer rates.[22] As international communications improve, the press will have an ever larger pool of unusual, and therefore more interesting, accident stories to write about. Why should we not expect an outcry from a public that reads about Love Canal, Times Beach, Alar, Chilean grapes laced with cyanide, and the leaflet of Villejuif,[23] whether or not such examples reflect meaningful danger?[24] (At the same time, how can one expect public reaction to potentially greater but more mundane problems, of which it is unaware?)

It is hard to make the normal human mind grapple with this inhuman type of problem. To change public reaction, one would either have to institute widespread public education in risk analysis or generate greater public trust in some particular group of experts or the institutions that employ them. The first alternative seems unlikely. The second, over the past thirty years, has not occurred. Ordinary, human, public perception, then, forms one element of the vicious circle.

Congressional Action and Reaction

A second element of the circle consists of Congressional reaction to perceived risk and to regulatory problems, which takes the form of detailed statutory instructions. Difficulties with these statutory provisions commonly arise out of language that, on its face, seems to grant the agency reasonable discretion, but which, through interaction with the administrative process, yields odd results. Consider, for example, CERCLA section 121(d), which says that EPA must clean up toxic waste sites to a condition that "at a minimum . . . assures protection of human health and the environment." The section goes on to specify that the "clean" site must also meet any other legal standard that is either (1) "applicable" or (2) "relevant and appropriate." It adds that such standards must include the "goals established under the Safe Drinking Water Act," but only if those goals are *relevant and appropriate* under the circumstances."[25]

This language sounds reasonable. The instruction to EPA to apply all "applicable" standards is perhaps redundant, for an "applicable" standard, by definition, applies. But what harm can a redundant instruction do? Moreover, concern about applying potentially unknown *other* standards, such as Safe Drinking Water Act goals, is mitigated by the qualifying phrase "relevant and appropriate."[26]

Nonetheless, such specific statutory language can create administrative difficulties, if applied to cleaning up a toxic waste dump like the *Ottati & Goss* site in southern New Hampshire. Safe Drinking Water Act goals often express ideal conditions that few actual drinking water systems can meet. Typical statutory goals, for example, may include "no carcinogens," a goal that, if taken literally, means not a single molecule of aflatoxin, red dye no. 2, or benzene, or, for that matter, not the tiniest microscopic particle of pepper, spinach, or mushroom. Such a goal would mean that, after a spill, IBM in California, say, would have to make the water its factory discharges far cleaner than the ocean or the bay into which it normally pours it (which is just what happened).[27]

At the same time, the "relevant and appropriate" language does not offer quite the escape hatch that its framers may have hoped. EPA, working through administrative procedures, creates norms, setting forth rules for typical cases, with exception procedures for unusual cases. The statute's language strongly suggests that Safe Drinking Water Act goals should be cleanup norms. It reinforces the views of those within EPA who may think this, and helps those with similar views outside EPA to bring lawsuits to enforce those views. Indeed, EPA officials may well know that Congress enacted this language in reaction to its concern that EPA was not "tough enough" in respect to cleanup; that Congress therefore may hold oversight hearings should EPA make too many exceptions; and that, given an individual legislator's political incentive to appear in interesting, positive news stories,[28] hearings are far more likely to mean criticism for leniency than for strictness.[29]

Once the goal becomes the norm, the path of least resistance is to follow it. To use the escape clause means added time, trouble, and procedure, including a potentially controversial public hearing. Administrators have a powerful incentive to apply these goals across the board, whether a spill takes place in a reservoir or in a swamp. Perhaps the cleanup effort I described in the New Hampshire waste dump cleanup case simply reflected an understandable administrative effort to apply rules—such as drinking water standards—across the board, without invoking exception procedures that might have meant further delay in an effort that nonetheless took ten years.

Occasionally a statutory provision goes further, itself setting a standard that seems unreasonably and pointlessly strict. The Delaney Clause,[30] applicable to food additives, and the "no migration of hazardous constituents" clause in the Solid Waste Disposal Act[31] seem to instruct the agencies not to permit addition, removal, or packaging of or by any substance that contains even a single molecule of an offending chemical, however large the cost or small the risk.

On other occasions, a statute will try directly to set the regulator's agenda. The 1984 Hazardous and Solid Waste Amendments, for example, list specific materials, such as dioxin, arsenic, cadmium, chromium, lead, mercury, nickel, selenium, and thelium, with great specificity—e.g., "dioxin-containing hazardous wastes numbered F020, F021, F022, and F023."[32] The amendments then instruct EPA to set standards for each of these substances within a particular time. Unless EPA does so, no one will be able to dispose of them in a landfill.[33] Clean Air Act Amendments also provide a strict statutory standard (to reduce risk to each individual to less than one in a million[34]—the risk of smoking two cigarettes in a lifetime) and provide similar statutory "hammers" designed to force EPA to promulgate standards for sources that fail to conform to the strict standard. The problem with this language is that it amounts to a set of shots in the dark. It tries to set and to control in detail EPA's cleanup agenda with directions that later experience may show to be inappropriate because they fail to achieve any reasonable policy goal.[35]

There are institutional reasons, however, why Congress may wish to write legislation of this kind. If the government is divided between the two major political parties, Congress may distrust the Executive Branch to carry out a more broadly worded instruction with sufficient vigor. Or, Congress may wish to indicate clearly that it is responsible for publicly desired strict regulation, whose ultimate costs, from a political perspective, may be less visible.[36] Individual legislators, in hearings from which legislation originates, know that they are more likely to receive visibility-raising publicity when they find a particular substance that may be dangerous; and they may then become committed publicly to its near eradication. The same incentives, again potentially leading to overly strict regulation, are operative in the well-publicized oversight hearings, which also help set an agency's regulatory agenda.[37]

Regardless, Congress is not institutionally well suited to write detailed regulatory instructions that will work effectively. For one thing, Congress enacts one statute at a time; it does not look at risk, or safety, or cancer prevention, as a set of related problems that might benefit from a unified approach. For another thing, legislation originates in different subcommittees, including several with overlapping jurisdiction, each of which must compete for political time and attention. Each subcommittee may consider the particular problems that it has studied as the most important, deserving a place at the head of the regulatory queue, whether or not dispassionate observers would reach the same conclusion. Finally, Congress is highly responsive to public opinion, as it ought to be. This means, however, that if the public finds it difficult to order risk priorities, Congress is also likely to find it difficult to write an effective agency agenda for addressing risk.[38] The second element of the vicious circle is connected to the first.

Uncertainties in the Technical Regulatory Process

The circle's third element consists of the uncertainties embedded in the regulatory process, and the assumptions the regulators must make in order to arrive at recommendations for actions despite those uncertainties. Predicting risk is a scientifically related enterprise, but it does not involve scientists doing what they do best, namely developing theories about how x responds to y, other things being equal. Rather, it asks for predictions of events in a world where the "other things" include many potentially relevant, rapidly changing circumstances, requiring the expertise of many different disciplines to reach a conclusion. A waste site evaluation, for example, may require knowledge of toxicology, epidemiology, meteorology, hydrology, engineering, public health, transportation, and civil defense, disciplines with different histories, different methods of proceeding, and different basic assumptions.[39] Moreover, where prediction involves a weak relationship, such as that between a small dose of a substance and a later cancer death, as well as long lead times, such as exposure for twenty years or more, it is difficult or impossible for predictors to obtain empirical feedback, which is necessary (for them as for all of us) to confirm or correct their theories. Scientists are happier looking for large differences in small populations over short periods than looking for small differences in large populations over long periods of time. To do the latter, they must make many simplifying assumptions that are often questionable.[40]

Many substance-risk regulatory assumptions arise from toxicology, the study of poisons. Like civil engineering, toxicology embodies as a disciplinary canon the importance of "erring on the safe side."[41] Toxicologists, in trying to determine the largest safe human dose of a suspect substance, have historically tended to divide by 100 the largest safe animal dose (called the Lowest Observed Effects Level).[42] Just as engineering will call bridges that meet the discipline's safety standards safe, and those that do not risky, so toxicology has tended to call doses that meet this "divided by 100 standard" safe. In more recent years, regulators have developed more refined standards, applied in a more complex regulatory system (and applied more frequently for small cancer risks than for other health risks). Yet one can find in many of that system's assumptions the shadow of toxicological "safety-first" canons.

Consider the enormous uncertainties, almost inevitably present, in any practical regulatory effort to carry out the four stages of risk assessment earlier described—identifying the hazard, relating response to dose, estimating exposure, and characterizing the risk. How is the risk assessor to determine the relation of a given disease with a small dose of the suspect substance? He must look either to statistical studies of human beings with the disease (epidemiological studies) or to studies of exposure to the substance in animals. Controlled epidemiological studies of the effects in humans of small doses over many years are prohibitively expensive (a definitive answer about saccharin would involve 100,000 subjects followed for nearly a generation).[43] Retrospective epidemiological studies (asking those with a given disease what substances they were exposed to) are cheaper, but still take considerable time, effort, and money, and sometimes raise more questions than they answer. (Were subjects and controls properly matched? Does a higher than average cancer rate reflect the effects of saccharin itself, or of other elements in the diet of saccharin users—who may, as a group, be overweight or better-off financially, or more likely to report the disease? Did cancer victims, understandably concerned about their disease more vividly recall the use of saccharin than their healthier "control" counterparts?)[44]

The more frequently used animal studies are often more uncertain.[45] The investigator applies a high dose of a supposed carcinogen to the animals; if they develop a higher than average number of tumors, the analyst tries to extrapolate backward to low doses in humans. What assumptions shall be made in doing so? What extrapolation model should be used? Risk analysts tend to use, for both animal and epidemiological studies, a linear model, which extrapolates backward on a straight line.[46] If, for example, a 5 percent saccharin diet causes tumors in 30 percent of all rats exposed (i.e., 300 per thousand), the model (to simplify) would indicate that one hundredth of the dose, a 5/100 of 1 percent saccharin diet, would cause tumors in one hundred times fewer rats, i.e., 3/10 of 1 percent of all rats (3 per thousand). Critics argue that to use such mathematical models is like saying "If ten thousand men will drown in ten thousand feet of water, then one man will drown in one foot of water," or "If dropping ten bottles off a ten-foot wall breaks all ten, then dropping ten bottles off a one-foot wall will break one."[47]

The critics are right, in that there is no consistent scientific rationale for assuming a linear relation between dose and response.[48] Some substances, such as cyanide, are proportionately as deadly in small doses as large ones; others, such as butter, are harmful only when consumed in large quantities; while still others, such as iodine, kill in high doses, are harmless in small doses, and in tiny doses are necessary for life. Science very often does not tell us which of these examples best applies. The human body may tolerate perfectly well dioxin exposures below a specific threshold; it may have certain chemical receptors that hold dioxin harmless, until the receptors' capacity is exceeded and dioxin is released into the body, with harmful consequences.[49] The carcinogenic effects of certain kinds of radiation may be determined more by the schedule of exposure than by the actual dose.[50] In respect to many regulated substances, the scientific answer to the question "Which extrapolation model?" is "We do not know." Nonetheless, regulators may use linear models for reasons of mathematical convenience rather than science.[51]

Unfortunately, ignorance about these issues is matched by their importance. The choice of a dose/response extrapolation model can make an enormous difference to how risky small doses of the substance appear to be.[52] Two scientifically plausible models for the risk associated with aflatoxin in peanuts or grain may show risk levels differing by a factor of 40,000.[53] OSHA, in trying to carry out the Supreme Court's mandate to find evidentiary support for its risk conclusion about low levels of benzene exposure, simply applied a linear model to high dose/response figures similar to those that had been long available. The linear model's critics would say that, given the large population of the United States, use of such a model too often produces a finding that a substance that kills a rat with large doses will kill some human being somewhere, almost however small the dose.[54]

Given the uncertainties and the importance of the matter at hand, what is the regulator to do?[55] With estimates that vary by such magnitudes, a simple retreat to the toxicological principle of erring on the side of safety will not solve the problem.[56]

There are other, similar problems. How shall the analyst report animal test results? Whatever dose/extrapolation model is used will probably yield a range of results, lying within bounds set by mathematical criteria designed to rule out simple coincidences. Shall the analysis report the lower bound of this range ("if all Americans eat five peanuts per year, *fewer than* one [zero] will die of cancer"), the upper bound ("no *more than* 80 will die"), a "most probable estimate midpoint," if there is one, within that range, or all of the above? Until now, risk analyses have tended to emphasize the upper bound (on "err on the side of safety" grounds), which may significantly overstate the problem.[57]

To what extent should the analyst assume, even in respect to high doses, that an animal resembles a human,[58] or, more generally, that experimental results from rats or mice can be extrapolated to humans?[59] Some scientists, noting that animal testing means exposing the animal to the highest dose that fails directly to injure the animal in certain defined ways, argue that the very size of this Maximum Tolerated Dose generates tumors. By killing large numbers of cells, it brings about quick cell regeneration, which entails a risk of cancer-causing mutations not present where fewer cells die more slowly over time.[60]

Others dispute this hypothesis and point to studies showing reasonably good correlations between animal studies and epidemiological studies of the same substances, suggesting that animal data may often be useful in evaluating carcinogenic risk to humans.[61] Still others point to obvious ways in which rats and mice may, or may not, resemble humans. Formaldehyde causes nasal cancer in rats but not mice; does this reflect the fact that rats, unlike mice and humans, breathe only through their noses?[62] Rats are smaller than humans; they do not live as long; they eat more grain (and thus ingest more aflatoxin) proportional to body weight;[63] they have certain internal organs that we lack (and vice versa);[64] they have chemical transporting pathways to internal organs that we may, or may not, share.[65] Regulators' assumptions sometimes "conservatively" overlook potentially relevant differences—by, for example, using results in whatever species proves most sensitive to a high dose of the test substance.[66] Other times, regulators' assumptions ignore risk-generating factors such as the existence of human pathways not found in a test animal through which a chemical might arrive at a particular organ.

Uncertainty also characterizes exposure estimates. Analysts may not know how many persons, across the nation, are exposed to different doses of different chemicals for different periods of time. They may suspect, but not know, that certain groups (such as workers at a particular factory) are exposed more than others. What exposure assumptions shall they use? In assessing individual risks EPA sometimes makes a strictly mechanical assumption that the individual is exposed to emissions at a point 200 meters from the factory, all day, every day, for 70 years.[67] OSHA assumes a factory worker exposed 8 hours per day, 5 days a week, 50 weeks per year, for 45 years.[68] Other agencies use such "conservative" assumptions as that householders spend 70 years in the same house (they spend 9, on average); that adults drink 2 liters of water per day (they drink 1.4 liters of all liquids); that half of all houses near toxic waste dumps contain children (remember the situation in the New Hampshire case), and so forth.[69]

If an agency uses these assumptions when calculating the risks run by individuals who are *maximally* exposed, they may be realistic; if it uses them to estimate effects on typical workers or citizens across the nation, they may be unrealistically conservative; if it uses them as "presumptions"—asking industry to come forward with proof of the contrary—they may, in practice, come to resemble the latter use. OMB argues that the agencies apply these assumptions too conservatively; it concludes that, taken together, they "often" overstate risks by factors of a thousand or even a million or more.[70] At the same time, even such assumptions sometimes can overlook special, much greater than average exposures—exposures via multiple pathways,[71] or exposures that pose special risks to those who also smoke or are also exposed to other chemicals.

The upshot is a system that may work well for assessing many large, serious risks, but where small risks are at issue it will generate results likely based on a host of controversial assumptions. Those assumptions often seem weighted in a conservative ("safety first") direction when applied to average or typical cases, because they rely on linear dose extrapolation models, upper confidence levels, most sensitive animal use, and average exposure assumptions.[72] At the same time, they may understate the possibilities of less usual combinations of circumstances that spell special danger—such synergisms as multiple substance exposures, multiple delivery pathways, unusually long exposures, and special sensitivities.[73] The analysis, in addition, may focus only upon cancer, perhaps putting to the side or investigating less thoroughly other potential harms, such as neurotoxicity, of less apparent concern to the public, and in respect to which it may also use less careful assumptions, such as the No Observable Effects Level.[74] How reasonable these various assumptions are, and how serious the limitations of the analysis may be, may vary from area to area, from substance to substance, from case to case. When errors arise, they do not offset each other (except by accident).[75]

The risk manager must take this analysis, and, in light of its conclusion, perhaps highly oversimplified, that a substance, say a pesticide, is a "known" or "suspect" carcinogen, ask such questions as (1) What will it cost to ban the substance (for example, what are the compliance costs, what are the costs of alternative pesticides)? (2) What benefits would we thereby lose (for example, the pesticide in question produces healthier, cheaper crops)? (3) Would a ban create other significant risks (for example, will farmers grow pest-resistant crops, say, "organic celery," with riskier natural carcinogens)? (4) What are the practicalities of enforcement (for example, the cost of measuring pesticide residues)? The answers to such questions also involve assumptions, guesswork, and subjectivity.

Before the 1970s, a regulator, faced with serious scientific uncertainty, and realizing that risk estimates rest upon assumptions whose reasonableness may vary from area to area, might simply have telephoned a trusted scientific friend to ask for an informal, off-the-record recommendation. Nowadays, current procedural rules aimed at fairness would probably stop such a phone call. Regulators now generally communicate with scientists more formally, through the medium of a public record. At the same time, scientists will often hesitate to state conclusions, publicly and on the record, that reach beyond scientifically acceptable evidence. They may say no more than "there is some evidence that . . . " or "there is no acceptable evidence that . . . ," although they also know that how they phrase their statement will inevitably affect the regulator's ultimate decision.[76] Thus the National Academy of Sciences panel may debate whether its saccharin report should say "available evidence does not indicate that saccharin is useful in weight control" or "scientific evidence does not permit assessment of the role that saccharin plays in weight control"; the difference (which may well affect public policy) is in the *form* of the statement, not its content. Of course, such subtle attention to communication may also lead to failure to communicate.

These uncertainties, knowledge gaps, default assumptions, guesses, and communications difficulties, all embodied in the technical regulatory process, spell trouble. They produce a system that, in respect to those average health risks that come to its attention, sometimes produces (for administrative, or canon-related, or mathematical reasons rather than scientific ones) conservative results that "err on the safe side." They also mean a system with limiting assumptions that threaten to pay less attention to more special, or synergistic, risks to health. Such a system, in respect to small risks, and with assumptions of varying reasonableness, can produce random results.

These problems also make it difficult for scientists and agency experts to reply to public claims that a substance is dangerous. When, for example, the press reported that EPA had begun to regulate the pesticide

EDB[77] and state regulators began to regulate tiny doses,[78] television news displayed a skull and crossbones along with pictures of chemical workers exposed to *pure* EDB.[79] Scientists had to respond truthfully that EDB in large doses is carcinogenic; some small risk may attach to small doses. The EPA administrator accurately added, "The truth is we don't know. We're operating in an area of enormous scientific uncertainty."[80] These answers are truthful given the uncertainties, but the word "uncertainty" itself implies risk; the denial therefore carries a kind of self-refutation that does not alleviate public concern. The EPA administrator continued: "We are operating with substances that the public is terribly afraid of. If they want absolute information, we can't give it to them."[81]

The very fact that the many assumptions required by uncertainties are not clearly derivable from science can make them a lightning rod for contending political forces. Regulatory bodies, after all, are politically responsive institutions, with boards, commissioners, or administrators appointed by the President, confirmed by the Senate, written about by the press, and, from time to time, summoned by Congressional committees to give public testimony.[82] Their agendas, within limits, respond to the public's demands. Their choices of default assumptions, to a degree, can respond to the desire of the President, Congress, Congressional staffs, interest groups, or the agencies themselves to appear especially careful to err on the safe side or alternatively to show sensitivity to economic costs.[83]

At the same time, regulators, seeking to create rules, must run a kind of gauntlet of critical reviewers, including staff at the Office of Management and Budget[84] and federal judges who judicially review agency actions at the request of any adversely affected person. Such reviews take time; they require non-expert judges to review highly technical matters on the basis of a record prepared by lawyers, not scientists; and they place a premium on compliance with a variety of procedural rules. Indeed, the very threat of judicial review has led agencies to adopt complex, time-consuming procedures both for making rules and for changing them.[85] The result is an agency that will sometimes hesitate to make rules[86] or to change them once adopted; consequently, rules become frozen in place and cannot readily adapt to changing scientific knowledge.[87]

Finally, these uncertainties, the consequent assumptions, and review rigidities, lead to a public and a Congress unlikely to disentangle the

complex combination of science, fact, value, and administration underlying the agency's risk conclusion—a public and a Congress that may
overemphasize a risk analysis's oversimplified "bottom line" while nonetheless suspecting that something about it is arbitrary. The reactions of
public and Congress are reinforced by those bottom-line numbers that
continue to be more concerned about tiny, widely diffused cancer threats,
and less concerned about other health-related matters.

The Vicious Circle

The three elements of the vicious circle—public perception, Congressional reaction, and the uncertainties of the regulatory process—
reinforce each other. Obviously, public perceptions influence Congress,
Congress (through press reports of its activities in particular) helps to
shape public perception, and both influence the response of agency
administrators to the problems they consider important.[88]

It is less obvious, but equally true, that the regulatory system's inherent
uncertainties make it more difficult for agencies to resist Congressional
or public efforts to set agendas and to manage particular results. Those
uncertainties, accompanied by scientific statements of doubt, along with
administrative practices such as default assumptions that differ among
agencies and among programs, give the appearance of subjective
decision-making. This appearance can encourage outside groups, such as
environmentalists who monitor agency performance, to try to generate
Congressional interest in particular agency decisions. Any such Congressional interest, in turn, will help to generate public interest, which tends
to move the particular problem at issue toward the top of the agency's
agenda ("random agendas") and creates more political pressure for a
stricter regulatory solution ("tunnel vision") or, particularly on less visible issues where industry groups provide effective countervailing political pressure, creates anomalous rulings ("inconsistency").

The circularity is reinforced by the fact that the more outside pressures
seem to control agency results, the less confidence the public will have
in the agency. The less confidence the public has in the agency, the
greater the perceived need for outside action, the greater the pressure
upon the agency to prove it has erred on the side of safety, and the greater
the tendency to adopt the public's risk agenda of the moment. Yet, as I

have argued, these latter tendencies, because of their irrational and counterproductive elements, will not help build public confidence.

Scientific uncertainties, together with "err on the safe side" scientific canons and default assumptions suggesting prevalent danger, may also help to convince environmentalists, press, and public that more should be done about known risks, particularly known carcinogenic risks, even when those risks are tiny. Such public pressure, in turn, may encourage Congress to enact standards or to supervise agencies by setting agency agendas and encouraging strong action in respect to those programs or substances that catch the public eye. Congressional reaction provokes further public concern. All of the above makes it more difficult for agencies to resist overkill and random agenda setting.

Given the uncertainties and regulatory methods, are the "tunnel vision" results surprising? Given Congressional statutes, likely agency reactions, and public pressures, should we not expect random risk-reducing agendas? Should we not expect regulators to react to what Congress, or the public, puts on their plates? Since Congress created different safety regulatory programs at different times, under different circumstances, with differing statutory language, administered by different agencies with different institutional environments employing different scientists from different disciplines, involving different publics with differing degrees of interest, why should we not expect to find inconsistent treatment of health and safety risks and inconsistent results (particularly when complex rule-creation and rule-review procedures tend to freeze old rules in place)?

By now, we have reached a kind of regulatory gridlock, whose mutually reinforcing causes tend to create agency regulation that "goes the last mile" to clean up "the last 10 percent," that creates random health (or safety) risk agendas, and that brings about inconsistent results among health and safety programs. Is it possible to cut this Gordian knot?

SOLUTIONS | 3

My suggestions for institutional change are designed not to change human nature, or the political nature of Congress, but to help break out of the "vicious circle." They are designed to attack the vicious circle at its weakest point, the regulatory link, and to change the circle's dynamics. They seek self-reinforcing institutional change, which will gradually build confidence in the regulatory system. My suggestions are based on several assumptions: The public wants better health and more safety overall. On balance, the public would like to have more risk reduction at current expenditure or similar risk reduction at less cost, i.e., it would like more "optimizing." The current hodgepodge of results does not reflect a public that really wants dirty Boston harbors and superclean swamps; rather, such policy priorities more likely reflect the psychological and practical difficulties of making risk decisions one substance at a time. Finally, I assume a kind of "general will"—a public that "really" wants an overall result that differs from its substance-specific preferences revealed on particular occasions.

Any practical, institutionally oriented solution must also take account of the extreme difficulty of changing human psychology, press reactions, or Congressional politics.[1] To speak of the need for improved communications with the public, or a more responsible press, or a more disciplined Congress is to call spirits from the vasty deep. One can call them, but will they come?

Nonetheless, it seems possible to suggest changes. Risk-related matters that enter the forum of public debate may have to pass political as well as technical tests for safety. But not every risk-related matter need become a public issue. A depoliticized regulatory process might produce better results, hence increased confidence, leading to more favorable public and Congressional reactions.

Non-Solutions

Let me begin my discussion of institutional solutions by describing briefly what will not work. I do not believe deregulation is the answer.[2] For one thing, some substances involve serious risks that must be regulated. The regulation of other substances, involving small risks at small doses, may seem totally unnecessary and may have safer, and no more expensive, alternatives, permitting agencies, through somewhat stricter regulation, to provide a little extra safety virtually cost-free. For another thing, deregulation does not address the failures of agencies to pursue more vigorously more serious environmental problems or to examine more systematically currently unexamined risks. Regardless, public demand for regulation is likely to continue, a demand that governments should not, and will not, ignore.[3]

Popular less restrictive alternatives, such as requiring labels on products,[4] or imposing taxes on risky products instead of setting standards,[5] offer more hope, but many such proposals also have serious shortcomings.[6] In respect to many labels, one must ask who reads them. To examine a printed warning from an aspirin package, with its many paragraphs of tiny print, is to wonder what the point of it is. Would the eagle-eyed reader who saw "risk of cancer: 1 in 100,000" know what that means? That reader does not want a warning; he wants to know what to do.[7] As a colleague once commented to me, given haphazard agency selections for testing, one might facetiously advise the consumer that the only safe substances are those labeled "danger"; at least we know that someone has tested them.

These criticisms may be unfair to some general, simplified labeling proposals, such as orange symbols for "mild risk" or green labels for "environmentally sound." They overlook tax proposals, such as taxes on environmental pollutants, which could apply to substances with low carcinogenic risk as well. Such proposals depend for their effectiveness on a practical, and political, ability to impose such taxes or affix such labels on appropriate products. They may constitute part of an administrative solution. But, even if labels and taxes help to alleviate some major health-risk problems, those problems seem likely to continue to call for more direct government intervention.

There are many obstacles to looking to Congress for significant help. As previously mentioned, Congressional committees and subcommittees with overlapping jurisdiction, political competition among members, legislation that proceeds one statute and subject matter at a time, distrust between branches that may be controlled by different political parties, a history of conflict arising out of what Congress saw as an Executive Branch effort to curtail environmental regulation, as well as the understandable Congressional tendency to respond quickly and directly to public perceptions, all work against the development of a more systematic, coordinated approach to regulating risks.[8]

The federal courts cannot do much better. Courts normally lack the power to require agencies to create systematically rational agendas. In fact, court requirements for action often simply reflect deadlines that Congress has written into different statutes;[9] enforcing such deadlines can distort agency agendas, by forcing the substance at issue to the head of the regulatory queue.

The Administrative Procedure Act permits the courts, normally considering one agency action at a time, to set aside those actions that are "arbitrary, capricious, an abuse of discretion."[10] The Fifth Circuit, as previously mentioned, set aside the EPA's decision concerning asbestos-containing materials.[11] Yet courts do not, and cannot, exercise this power very often.[12] In general courts are no more able—indeed they are less able than Congress—to consider agency agendas as a whole and to set priorities.[13]

Courts are aware that what seems unreasonable to a judge may not seem so to a regulator. The institutions are very different. Regulators must make "legislative-type" decisions, the merits of which depend upon finding, or prying, out important general facts about the world; they work in what is sometimes a politically charged environment; they may need to seek compromise solutions acceptable to warring private groups; they must reach a practical, administrable result that, on balance, will help achieve a statute's general public-interest goal. Judges must reach decisions that are fair, the merits of which depend upon the relevant legal norm and a record, prepared by lawyers, that need not contain all relevant facts about the world; they must reach their decisions without further factual investigation;[14] and they must do so within the context of a crowded docket.[15] Given these differences, a compromise solution that a regulator considers reasonable, for practical administrative reasons, may not seem rational to a judge, who must view that decision in the light of the statute, prior cases, and a notion of "good reason" more directly oriented toward the merits.[16]

Moreover, court decisions automatically generate legal precedents and legal rules. A legal rule that flows from a court decision overturning a particular action as arbitrary will sometimes help produce more rational results. But it may also lead the agency to turn to other, less fair, more complicated ways to achieve its objectives. For example, after the Fifth Circuit overturned the Consumer Product Safety Commission's formaldehyde rule, in *Gulf South*,[17] the Commission could achieve a comparable result simply by recalling formaldehyde-containing products, without benefit of an agency rule.[18]

The court's decision may also create unforeseen procedural difficulties. The Fifth Circuit, for example, overturned EPA's rule banning asbestos brake linings for the reason, inter alia, that EPA had not adequately considered the "alternatives"—that is, other ways to combat risks from asbestos.[19] As the Supreme Court has held, regulators should consider alternatives. But must there be thorough consideration of every alternative in every case? Sometimes the alternative consequences (costs/loss of benefits/risk) are obvious; sometimes it is obvious that lengthy investigation of an alternative will not yield significant additional relevant knowledge. Yet a judicial decision that says "consider alternatives" may be wielded as a precedent by advocates in later cases. It may lead the agency to establish procedures to consider thoroughly *all* alternatives in *every* case. The result may be lengthy, complicated disputes about alternatives, often entailing considerable unproductive delay.[20]

Aside from precedential effects, an adverse court decision typically means a remand, which, as in the benzene case, may lead to several more years of "corrective rulemaking proceedings" (as Richard Merrill calls them) to reach basically similar results.[21]

Courts understand these considerations. They therefore hesitate to call agency decisions irrational and set them aside.[22] Recent Supreme Court authority reinforces their hesitancy.[23] Moreover, the crowded state of judicial dockets offers a highly practical reason why judges will not, and probably should not, devote the considerable time and effort needed to review a several-thousand-page agency record, informed by a thorough understanding of the substance of risk-related regulatory problems, in order to see whether or not that agency determination was arbitrary.

Courts also administer a system of tort law which discourages the negligent production of risky substances by forcing producers (or their insurers) to compensate those whom they injure. That system, however, leaves the determination of "too much risk" in the hands of tens of thousands of different juries who are forced to answer the question not in terms of a statistical life, but in reference to a very real victim needing compensation in the courtroom before them. The result is a system much criticized for its random, lottery-like results and its high "transaction costs" (i.e., legal fees) which eat up a large fraction of compensation awards.[24] Whatever its merits and problems, I do not believe the tort system can serve as a substitute for government regulation.

The Characteristics of a Solution

Neither the courts nor Congress seem likely to provide real solutions to the problems of risk regulation. Major nonregulatory alternatives, deregulation, taxes, labeling, or greater public participation seem insufficient. Is it possible to find administrative help within the Executive Branch? Our problems are essentially problems of good government. Is there then a better-government or bureaucratic solution to the problems posed?

There are strong reasons for believing that an answer does lie in that direction.[25] I shall describe a possible change in administrative organization that is not a cure-all, nor a definitive answer, but, I believe, is a constructive approach. Like more radical changes, such as the creation of OMB itself (and perhaps like the creation of the Senior Executive Service),[26] its aim is to help to realize the hope for effective government implicit in any civil service able to attract honest, talented, and qualified administrators.

The suggestion has two parts: (1) establishment of a new career path that would provide a group of civil servants with experience in health and environmental agencies, Congress, and OMB; and (2) creation of a small, centralized administrative group, charged with a rationalizing mission, whose members would embark upon this career path. Such a proposal is likely to engender objections that the proposal sounds undemocratic, elitist, ineffective, politically unfeasible, and without any practical means of implementation. Before considering those objections, however, I wish to describe the essential characteristics of such a group, how it might draw on certain positive attributes of bureaucracies, the nature of its specific mission, and several examples of related institutional experience.

The discussion in the first two chapters suggests that the design of any new administrative group would have to incorporate five features. First, the group must have a specified risk-related *mission*—not the mission of "total safety" or "zero risk," or "maintaining economic productivity," but the mission of building an improved, coherent risk-regulating system, adaptable for use in several different risk-related programs; the mission of helping to create priorities within as well as among programs; and the mission of comparing programs to determine how better to allocate resources to reduce risks.

Second, the group must have *interagency jurisdiction.* Such jurisdiction is needed to bring about needed transfers of resources, say from toxic waste to vaccination or prenatal care; otherwise, efforts to overcome resource misallocation would remain somewhat theoretical, rather like discussions about transferring money spent on aircraft carriers to health care.[27] Without such interagency jurisdiction, the group would find it difficult to overcome the tendencies of separate agencies simply to compromise differences through a single meeting leading to a single rule determined administratively rather than scientifically, as when EPA, CPSC, and FDA recently ironed out their rat-to-man "comparative body weight" versus "comparative surface area" disagreement simply by choosing a number—body weight raised to the 3/4 power—that split the difference.[28] Without interagency jurisdiction, the group would find itself limited in its ability to find examples of comparable risk-related problems in different areas which it could use in building its system, to suggest priorities among programs, and to look for potentially creative ways to put health resources to work more effectively.

Third, the group must have a degree of *political insulation* to withstand various political pressures, particularly in respect to individual substances, that emanate from the public directly or through Congress and other political sources. At a minimum, a group's members must enjoy civil service protection.

Fourth, the group must have *prestige*. That prestige must both attract, and arise out of an ability to attract, a highly capable staff. A capable staff is one that understands science, some economics, administration, possibly law, and has the ability to communicate in a sophisticated way with experts in all these fields.

Fifth, the group must have the *authority* that will give it a practical ability to achieve results. Such authority may arise in part out of a legal power to impose its decisions. But it may also arise through informal contacts with line agency staffs, out of its perceived knowledge and expertise, out of "rationalizing" successes that indicate effectiveness, and out of the public's increased confidence that such successes may build.

In summary, my proposal is for a specific kind of group: mission oriented, seeking to bring a degree of uniformity and rationality to decision making in highly technical areas, with broad authority, somewhat independent, and with significant prestige. Such a group would make general and government-wide the rationalizing efforts in which EPA is currently engaged.[29] Let me now turn to why the creation of such a group might help.

Drawing upon the Virtues of Bureaucracy

The group I have in mind, composed of civil servants who are following the proposed career path, would draw strength from its ability to harness several virtues inherent in many administrative systems: rationalization, expertise, insulation, and authority.

1. *Rationalization*. Bureaucracies rationalize the problems and processes with which they work, allowing them to develop systems. For example, gradually over several decades, bureaucracies charged with setting rates for electricity, communications, and transportation have developed a complex but fairly uniform system of "cost of service ratemaking." That system does not consist simply of rules and regulations. Rather, the rules are accompanied by standards, practices,

guidelines, prototypes, models, and informal procedures, all shaped to some extent by a general goal (that of replicating a competitive market-place) but more directly guided by goals internal to the system (efficiency, fairness, fair return on investment). The system solves roughly similar problems in roughly similar ways irrespective of the particular regulatory program or regulated industry at issue.[30]

The problems of health and safety risk regulation could well benefit from the development of a similar system. Such a system would recognize differences between, say, unusually high risks to specially placed individuals and risks to a general population. It would neither reduce all lives saved to a common dollar-value, nor claim incommensurable differences among different health programs and circumstances. Such a system would compare experience under different programs to create a uniform approach, while embodying that approach in models, examples, and paradigms that permit local variation. Ratemaking problems are somewhat simpler, yet they suggest a parallel.

2. *Expertise.* Bureaucracies develop expertise in administration, but also in the underlying subject matter. They normally understand that subject matter at least well enough to communicate with substantive experts, to identify the better experts, and to determine which insights of the underlying discipline can be transformed into workable administrative practices, and to what extent. A unified group charged with developing a system for addressing health risk regulation might bring together people familiar with science, risk analysis, economics, and administration—expertise that now is divided among different agencies, such as EPA and OMB.

3. *Insulation.* A civil service automatically offers a degree of insulation or protection both from politics and from public opinion. Of course, tenure rules tend to insulate its members, to some extent, from the force of public criticism. More important, administrators of a system can rationalize or justify particular results in particular cases in terms of the system's rules, practices, and procedures. Just as a doctor justifies a dose of bitter medicine by reference to medical theory and practice that indicate it will help the patient, so regulators explain and justify highly unpopular individual decisions, such as a decision that means a significant rate increase for the public. They do so through reference to the rules and practices of a system that, considered as

a whole, helps the public by keeping rates within reason. Use of a coherent, well-worked-out system changes the focus of political questions. It becomes more difficult simply to ask, "Isn't this specific result terrible?" The relevant question becomes, "Is this a good *system;* and, if so, does the system generate this particular result?" Bureaucratic solutions, if sound and coherent, resting on well-constructed comparisons among different substances, offer administrators the promise of a modest increase in independence, through greater insulation from public criticism of individual decisions.

4. *Authority.* A bureaucratic solution offers the hope of creating authoritative decisions that may, in turn, help break the vicious circle. Respect for decisions as authoritative is not easy to create in this era of political distrust, an era that since 1970 has seen Americans' confidence in virtually every institution—government, business, the press (but, surprisingly, not the military)—plummet (see Figure 4),[31] and an era in which different political parties control Congress and the Executive Branch. Still, it seems to me that public respect depends not only upon the perception of public participation but also, in part, upon an organization's successful accomplishment of a mission that satisfies an important societal need. (Consider the rebound of confidence in the military during the 1980s.) If that is so, the authority or legitimacy of a particular regulatory action depends in part upon its technical sophistication and correctness, and in part upon its conformity with the law, and both parts help to determine the extent of public confidence in the regulator.

Insofar as a systematic solution produces technically better results, the decision will become somewhat more legitimate, and thereby earn the regulator a small additional amount of prestige, which may mean an added small amount of public confidence. Any such increase in trust may encourage greater legislative respect. As a central bureaucratic group attains a degree of prestige and develops contacts, Congressional committees may begin to ask it for advice in drafting legislation, thereby helping further to rationalize risk-regulation programs and expenditures. Congress might delegate it additional or broader regulatory authority. That authority may increase the agency's prestige, making it easier to attract better-trained personnel, who may in turn do a better technical job, which in turn may generate increased public confidence. These tendencies, even if only gradual, point in the right direction.

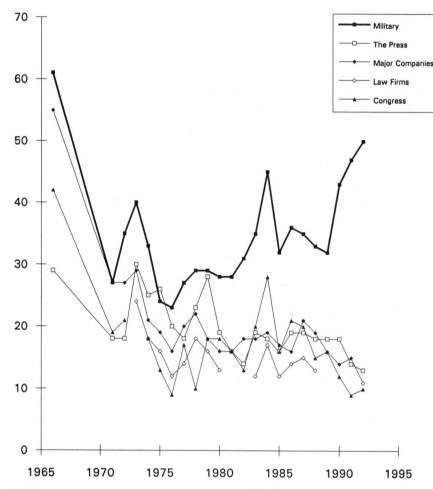

Figure 4. Percent of respondents answering "a great deal of confidence" when asked if they would have "a great deal of confidence, only some confidence, or hardly any confidence" in people running the institution. *Source:* Louis Harris and Associates, Inc., Harris Poll, March 22, 1992.

A Reformed Mission

My second reason for optimism is that one can fairly easily draft a specific agenda that would take advantage of these inherent bureaucratic virtues. A centralized administrative group, charged with helping to develop a uniform system, could usefully draw upon the experience of different agency efforts to achieve the same goal (health-risk reduction) in different circumstances, in several ways.

First, it could usefully try to make explicit, and more uniform, controversial assumptions that agencies now, implicitly and often inconsistently, use in reaching their decisions. For example, regulators should investigate carefully in order to avoid actions that kill more people than they save. Comparative program experience is likely to suggest more uniform relevant standards.[32] To take another example, is there some *de minimis* level of risk below which any program ought to consider a substance safe?[33] Is there some level of expenditure beyond which a program should not go in its efforts to save a single statistical life? And are these two questions related? To work out a *de minimis* standard involves considering both the extent to which small doses of a substance pose risks to the population at large (for example, "substance x threatens 100 additional deaths across the nation"), and the extent to which exposure poses certain special risks to particular individuals (for example, "only 200 people are exposed to substance x, but each of them has a fifty-fifty chance of death"), considered in light of costs, broadly defined—in that tiny costs may warrant stricter standards aimed at tiny risks, and vice versa. Currently, permitted risk levels vary widely—even ranging between one in ten thousand and one in a million within a single proposal—both between and within programs and agencies, against a vague legislative background whose statutes simply announce the criteria of "acceptable," "safe," or "significant" level of risk, typically tempered by concerns of economic and technical feasibility expressed in vague, general terms.[34] The *de minimis* problem is complex but it does not defy efforts to create a more uniform, commonsense standard, if only a presumptive standard that would permit exceptions, or even if only a set of examples of frequently found tradeoffs and acceptable risk levels that would help agencies develop their own rules.[35]

Second, a central group could make conscious efforts to draw upon scientific and technical work found outside the government. Some outside experts, for example, have developed systematic and sophisticated methods of factoring different kinds of uncertainty into risk analyses; others have developed methods for assessing how particular communities value different health-risk reduction programs.[36] The central group, working with existing Science Advisory Boards, could select and disseminate such work, which could help inform the judgmental risk-regulatory process in much the same way that good econometric models inform, but do not determine, judgmental "rate of return" decisions.[37]

Third, a central group could help develop models that aim to achieve higher-quality analysis and better results. Models build uniform systems, while recognizing that different circumstances may call for different treatment. Exposures of specially sensitive populations, for example, or exposures through multiple pathways, or dose extrapolation models with thresholds, will sometimes, as a matter of commonsense, be highly relevant to a regulatory judgment, and sometimes not. To create uniform, multi-program rules in advance about such matters can provoke heated but unenlightening debate; yet for each agency to go its own way means serious inconsistency. Models or prototypes or examples, flagging key assumptions and providing options at key points, can produce a system with uniform aims which is also adaptable.

Models based upon interagency experience could help regulators decide how to find some kind of natural regulatory stopping place, short of zero risk or the destruction of an industry, which does not depend upon the regulator's subjective reaction to the facts of an individual case. The models might use comparisons that would themselves create, without specifically defining, standards that the human mind can grasp, that limit arbitrary action, and that achieve consistency.

Models and examples might explain how usefully to "unpack" crude risk-assessment numbers and simple qualitative conclusions through comparisons that illuminate the nature of relevant uncertainties (e.g., substance A is like B in respect to x, but like C in respect to y).[38] They might illustrate the use of "sensitivity analysis" to explain how technical conclusions change in reaction to small changes in default assumptions; they might explain different kinds of uncertainty; they might depict ranges of estimates, rather than relying upon, say, "upper confidence levels"; they might illustrate different ways in which an agency can take account of the benefits that a substance provides, the direct costs of removing it, and the risks that accompany alternatives.[39] All this is to suggest a need for a system that provides neither a single set of rules nor a myriad of approaches, that simplifies but recognizes the need for a few major variations, and that guides through standard, paradigm, and example, but does not directly command.

Fourth, the centralized group might create a "risk agenda" that helps to prioritize different programs, and different activities within programs, and that looks for tradeoffs among programs that will lead overall to improved health or safety. It might, for example, look for practical ways to settle some toxic waste dump cases, thereby obtaining funds that might be used to help pay for vaccinations, or prenatal care, or mammograms; or it might look for practical ways to charge "low-risk-substance" fees that are then used for similar purposes. It might, in other words, look for ways to reallocate, transfer, or combine health resources so that they perform more effectively.

Fifth, the group might consider the likely risk-related impact of future scientific changes. Suppose, for example, that medical research identifies particular groups of persons genetically predisposed to develop cancer when exposed to certain chemicals.[40] Society should not ignore their special plight. Yet it may prove nearly impossible, and sometimes inordinately expensive, to grant them a "right" to the lowest possible risk and then limit society's use of chemicals to which they specially react. It might well be more effective to provide them with special counseling that includes information about how to avoid exposure to the carcinogens to which they are particularly susceptible. Problems of special risks to a limited population—where risks to the general population may be small, where costs of ordinary regulatory solutions may be high, and where alternative ways to lower special risks might be found—resemble in kind but not degree the problems many regulators now face.[41] It is this kind of "future-oriented" problem that a group such as I propose might find on its agenda.

Having found the links among the three elements of the "vicious circle" (public, Congress, and the regulatory process) virtually forged in iron, and aware of no obvious practical way to affect the first two elements, I am looking for a way to recast the third element to help us harness the inherent virtues of civil service to bring about improved performance. The discussion so far has suggested certain major characteristics of a bureaucracy that, in principle, match the needs described earlier. A bureaucracy's rationalizing tendencies match the need for consistency through system-building and prioritizing; a bureaucracy's use of expertise matches the need for technically related regulatory improvement; a bureaucracy's insulation matches the need for protection from the vicissitudes of public opinion based on a single substance or on a single issue; and a successful bureaucracy can begin to build public confidence in its systems, thereby making its results more authoritative. The discussion has also suggested a fairly specific administrative agenda that seems capable of implementation, which would help to achieve the results that these bureaucratic virtues promise.

Examples

Consider several examples that may help clarify what I have in mind. Single agencies have made serious efforts to inject better science into the regulatory process. In 1974, EPA created its Science Advisory Board (SAB), staffed by experts from academia, industry, and public interest groups, to strengthen the scientific basis of its policymaking. Congress ratified this move with legislation in 1978, and has since given the SAB increased responsibility and independence within EPA.[42] The EPA has also come to use more specialized advisory committees, both internal and independent. Those who have studied the work of these committees find that they have led to significant improvements, a result that is tied to the facts that members are senior scientists, that members remain on committees for a fairly long period of time, and that consultation is often private and nonadversarial.[43] Single agencies have also tried to rationalize and prioritize different agency programs. EPA has begun to do so.[44] The Department of Health and Human Services has created a subagency, called the Agency for Health Care Policy Research, that looks for ways to allocate health protection resources more effectively. A central administrative group would bring to such efforts an increased ability to make interagency comparisons, priorities, and transfers, an increased capacity to obtain multidisciplinary expertise, increased insulation from local politics, and perhaps a greater incentive to succeed in its rationalizing mission.

The Executive Branch already contains groups that seek to harmonize the activities of different agencies. OMB's Office of Information and Regulatory Affairs, for example, reviews regulatory agendas and major regulations that line agencies intend to propose. OIRA's basic job is to bring about the kind of rationalization I have described.[45] Indeed, OIRA is the lineal descendant of efforts by Presidents Nixon, Ford, and Carter to achieve greater coordination within the huge Executive Branch, efforts embodied in the Council on Wage and Price Stability (under Ford), the Regulatory Affairs Review Group (under Carter), and various executive directives mandating coordinated or at least consistent evaluation of proposed regulations.[46] OIRA, however, has only about forty professional staff members. Its staff consists primarily of policy analysts who are trained in economics rather than science. And the chief source of its authority, the connection through OMB to the White House, has provoked charges that it wields undue political influence that has aggravated friction with line agency staffs and undermined public confidence.[47]

More important, OIRA differs from a line agency such as EPA, whose work it reviews, in the training of its staff members (economics vs. environmentally related sciences), its mandate (cost control vs. reduced risks), its approaches to problems (reduction to a single [dollar] metric vs. circumstance-specific results), and its susceptibility to political influences (presidential vs. Congressional). Given these differences, it is surprising that the tensions that now exist have not been greater.

OMB, acting through other administrative units, has the power to control most line agencies in respect to budget or to agency positions on proposed legislation. But OMB does not enjoy the necessary mandate to coordinate, nor does it have the substantive expertise to carry out a reform agenda.[48] The Office of Science Advisor to the President has considerable scientific expertise, but that office, and others like it, lacks size, experience with the administrative detail that accompanies specific program implementation, and direct authority. The President's Council of Economic Advisors, though involved in regulation-rationalizing activities, has similar constraints, and has primarily an economic, rather than a regulatory mission. Some of the economically oriented approaches to regulation it has supported, such as environmental taxes and marketable "pollution rights," may prove a useful contribution.[49]

A less formal but frequently used centralized administrative device to help achieve coordination is an ad hoc task force that brings together staff members from line agencies (and perhaps representatives from OMB, OIRA, or the Science Advisor) to discuss common problems and to write a report. Indeed, such task forces are now meeting within the Executive Branch, trying to work out common approaches to risk regulation.[50] Such efforts, however, typically suffer from their ad hoc status. The number of individuals involved is often small, and they may have other duties and responsibilities. The ad hoc groups rarely exist long enough, or have sufficient authority, to see that their recommendations are implemented or to adapt or revise those recommendations as different program demands and changing circumstances may require. Their short lifespan also prevents them from applying lessons learned in one program to future regulatory problems.

Under the Carter Administration the heads of line agencies—EPA, OSHA, CPSC, FDA, and others—met once a week to coordinate approaches in an interagency regulatory liaison group.[51] This group, however, had only a small staff and no independent ability to investigate or resolve the larger problems I have been discussing.

Other nations offer examples of far more powerful coordinating mechanisms. In France, for example, line agency work is coordinated, to a degree, by substantively oriented *inspecteurs de finance* and the more legally oriented Conseil d'Etat. Most members of the Conseil are recruited from among the top graduates of the prestigious Ecole Nationale d'Administration; others enter laterally from elsewhere in the civil service, in midcareer. In its judicial role, the Conseil reviews the lawfulness of any challenged administrative decree, regulation, or administrative action. Its members may also participate in the Conseil's second, important consultative role, offering advice to the ministries (and to the council of ministers), and reviewing in advance proposed decrees, rules, and regulations (some of which in this country would take the form of legislation) both for legality and for technical quality. Subsequently, their civil service careers will lead them through different, typically high-level line agency positions, say, in the treasury, in an economic planning agency, in a nationalized industry, or even in an embassy abroad. A successful career may eventually lead back to the Conseil, to the highly prestigious position of *conseiller*, a type of judge and advisor to the executive who reviews the "administrative lawfulness" of government actions and proposed regulations.

Each member of the Conseil's staff is thus technically well trained in administration, in administrative laws, rules, and procedures, and (depending upon individual experience) in some substantive subject matter. Prior experience provides many of its members with a general, perhaps a global, view of governmental programs. Its central administrative location (outside any specific line agency), the universal application of its administrative law expertise, and its consultative function help it to transmit knowledge and experience across program boundaries. Its prestige, the influence and contacts of its members, its formal power (the power to review agency rules for administrative legality, consistency, and drafting quality, and to set unlawful agency actions aside), and its power to influence (to review in advance and to advise ministries about regulations and policies) give the Conseil considerable practical ability to shape and sometimes directly to control outcomes.[52]

Of course, America is not France; nor are the substantive problems of risk regulation exactly the same as the problems of administrative regularity, legality, and efficacy that typically face the Conseil d'Etat. Nonetheless, it is worth considering the attributes that make such a centralized administrative organization successful and considering whether some of those attributes might be transferable to a parallel organization in the United States. After all, the "circulating career path" for persons who will eventually become high-level executives is not unique to France (the U.S. Forest Service uses it to great advantage,[53] as does American business); nor are efforts to bring together top administration and technical knowledge (recall EPA's use of Science Advisory Boards); nor are centralized review mechanisms (OMB and OIRA). One might imagine a centralized American civil service institution consciously designed to attain prestige (reflecting recruitment, administrative rank, previous success, tradition, power, and perhaps pay), to develop among its staff members practical experience in line agencies as well as at the "center," to maintain contacts (in part developed through that experience), and to wield some degree of power (both to persuade and to control).

Suppose a special group was created within OMB that offered its staff members a special civil service career path, leading through line agencies such as EPA, FDA, OSHA, and also passing through Congress, where the civil servant could join a Congressional committee staff, leading back to the OMB group, with the more successful staff member perhaps becoming Science Advisor to the President, or Member of the Council of Economic Advisors, or Director of OMB, or Judge on the U.S. Court of Appeals in Washington, D.C. This career path would provide the civil servant with experience in policy analysis, finance, substantive line work (in, for example, health regulation), legislation, and law. It would also help the corps of such civil servants develop a network of contacts throughout the federal government, which in turn would help to expand its influence. A cadre of individuals, following such a career path, would obtain experience in several different programs, agencies, and branches of government. A central unit within OMB, staffed with such individuals, might be given the kind of rationalizing mission that I earlier described; and, with such a staff, it might find its work more readily accepted within the line agencies than does OIRA.[54]

The immediate source of this group's power might lie in its assumption of OIRA's present mandate to review line agencies' proposed rules and regulations, augmented by its missions to rationalize risk regulation and seek tradeoffs. This comes close to suggesting an enhanced OIRA, a concept that environmentalists might find threatening. But staffing an augmented OIRA with scientifically or substantively trained experts, working alongside policy analysts and economists, could mute potential conflicts between OIRA and line agencies.

Even very modest success for such a group might lead to expanded authority. For example, the Council of Economic Advisors' primary responsibility for considering, modifying, and proposing economically oriented regulatory supplements (such as taxes, or marketable rights, or "risk budgets") might naturally gravitate toward such a group, finding itself included among the group's responsibilities. Perhaps such a group would begin to consider whether proposed rules, regulations, or major agency actions are "arbitrary, capricious, an abuse of discretion"—a legal authority that would bring with it enormous power. Indeed, a civil service group, better equipped to investigate general, science-related facts than a court, and operating in the present legal world of "restrained" judicial review, might find the practical scope of that authority growing, gradually supplanting the (additional, same-standard) review by a court and thereby transforming the group into a kind of administrative court along European lines.

Objections

Now let me turn to five major objections that could be made to my proposal for a new, centralized bureaucratic group.

1. *It is undemocratic.* It may be objected that the proposal would grant too much power to the central Executive Branch at the expense of Congress; it is undemocratic because it disregards Jefferson's advice not to "take" power from the people but to "inform their discretion."[55]

A moment's thought, however, reveals that the proposal takes no power from Congress. The Executive Branch currently exercises the power that any such group would possess, but it does so in a disorganized, somewhat random way. Chaos is not democracy; to organize rationally the exercise of power may mean its better, but not its greater, exercise.

Success, of course, might lead Congress to delegate to the Executive Branch broader regulatory authority than it has at present. But any Congressional decision to broaden statutory mandates would have to reflect a democratically made judgment that the broader delegation would bring about results more consistent with the public's basic health and safety demands. Broad delegation is not itself undemocratic; the public often recognizes that such delegation is essential to achieve an important general public goal, say, the regulation of securities. Congress does not write statutes that direct the battle movements of individual Army tank corps, nor could the Army win battles if it did so. For reasons I have mentioned, to achieve the public's broader health and safety goals may require forgoing direct public control of, say, individual toxic waste dumps.

Is any such diminution of the power of individual Congressional subcommittees (or their members' constituents) to control particular substance-specific or place-specific outcomes itself undemocratic? To the contrary. The power of local groups or interests to control decisions that affect more than one Congressional district is itself not particularly democratic; parochialism is not democracy. Indeed, a "pessimistic democrat," such as the Rousseau of *The Social Contract,* would argue that the only viable form of democracy is one in which the people make the simple but vital choice of approving or disapproving the proposals of a "lawgiver."[56] Put in more contemporary terms, the existence of a single, rationalizing group of administrators can thus facilitate democratic control, for it would reduce a mass of individual decisions to a smaller number of policy choices, publicize the criteria used to make those choices, and thereby make it easier for Congress, or the public, to understand what the Executive Branch is doing and why. Both Congress and the public could therefore more easily hold Executive Branch decision makers responsible, and a yes or no vote would more meaningfully express the wishes of the voter.[57] To systematize, to create clear lines of authority, to facilitate the assignment of responsibility is to empower the public. Representative democracy is not undemocratic.

2. *Selection of group members is elitist.* The best defense against a charge of elitism is to point out that the word is not an argument but simply a pejorative label. One can equally well apply a different label to the principle of recruitment, such as "the search for quality and competence." Is it not worth trying to recruit highly qualified people into government? Is protecting the public health not a worthwhile use of their time? In conjunction with adequate levels of compensation and working conditions at the higher levels of the civil service,[58] the career path that I have sketched could reasonably be expected to attract such people through its promise of increased authority, prestige, and potential accomplishment.

3. *It would be ineffective.* The most serious criticism is that proposals of this kind do not accomplish anything. They simply amount to reshuffling administrative boxes, perhaps creating a few new bureaucratic bottles out of which pours the same old, bad wine. In reply, I can only point to the nature of the administrative task, the specific agenda, the list of necessary attributes, and the inherent characteristics of the kind of organization described. The centralized administrative group in several respects offers a kind of "middle ground." It is meant to know about many different regulatory programs, yet have the mission of creating unifying models that can be adapted to suit different regulatory contexts. It is meant to have a staff that understands science and economics, yet, by rotating through a number of assignments, learns enough about Congressional politics and high-level administration so that it does not become narrowly expert. The staff is meant to work with Congressional statutes and regulatory rules, yet with a mission (and experience) that should prevent it from becoming overly "proceduralist" or "lawyer-like." It is meant to reach beyond a single agency both because risk regulation itself does so (consider OSHA and FDA, as well as EPA) and because, by doing so, it may imaginatively make connections that otherwise it might not see. It is meant as an alternative that helps to avoid both local

program-oriented agency/subcommittee/interest-group fragmentation and substance-by-substance, or regulation-by-regulation, revisions based upon overly simplistic "dollars-per-life-saved" evaluations by a cost-oriented reviewing body. Examples from more centralized civil services suggest (though they do not prove) that this list of objectives is not Utopian.

Consider how these advantages might help this new institution deal with the three major problems discussed in Chapter 1. The solution to the problem of unwarranted costs to protect nonexistent "dirt-eating children" is simply to stop short of the unnecessary, unproductive attempt to remove "the last 10 percent" of risk. Why would a centralized administrative group make it easier, or more likely, for EPA's New Hampshire lawyers to say that 90 percent cleanup is enough? After all, EPA itself, or a bureau within EPA, or the lawyers themselves, might also have said enough is enough.

For one thing, a centralized group of administrators with a specific reform mission might produce a technically better governing or guiding rule, or presumption, or principle, or model or set of practices, that would help local administrators know when to stop. Remember that "the last 10 percent" is simply shorthand for "going too far." The New Hampshire EPA lawyers need to know specifically what to do. To examine a little gasoline mixed with New Hampshire dirt does not tell them (nor does the toxic waste program or statute tell them) how clean is clean enough. Properly to answer the tens of thousands of such individual questions arising within a myriad regulatory programs requires a system that guides local answers. To build such a system requires examining program objectives, measured against available resources, in light of a host of scientific and administrative capacities and limitations.

A centralized administrative group, in developing such a system, has many advantages that more local groups may lack. Its staff has experience in different programs and a mix of technical and administrative skills, and is placed in an institution without a single-minded goal (of "no risk," or "economic productivity"). The group's base of information automatically extends beyond a single program or a handful of programs. Like EPA, the group would work with Science Advisory Boards. It could readily draw upon technical and scholarly work by independent investigators, such as studies of how to use citizen "focus groups" to help assign value to risk reduction, and estimates of the relation among increased expenditure, diminished economic productivity, and health. In the area of rate-setting regulation, such interaction among several agencies working on similar problems and outside experts has produced technically better answers to similarly difficult judgmental questions, such as "What is a fair rate of return on capital?" A centralized group might consciously try to replicate this interactive experience.

For another thing, as I have previously mentioned, the existence of any such government-wide system would make it easier, hence more likely, for EPA's central or local administrators (say, those concerned with cleanup of wetlands in New Hampshire) to stop short of "the last 10 percent," because following a system—even one that guides rather than dictates—offers the local administrators insulation and protection from criticism. They can answer the locally posed question, "Is our swamp clean now?" with, "Yes, the swamp is clean; the risks are insignificant; and national technical (system-based) standards say that is so."

Further, the centralized group, by comparing program experience, may find better answers to special problems, such as those posed by program-specific statutory language—say, language that seems to require cleanup to the point of "zero risk." Statutory language is rarely that precise; rather, it almost always leaves a linguistic loophole, if only the meaning of the word "safety," which depends, in part, upon context. A centralized group might develop consistent ways of interpreting statutory language, which, in the context of an overall system, might avoid wasteful results while better achieving Congress's overall health and safety objectives.

Finally, a centralized administrative group may better be able to develop systematic methods for capturing some of the resources saved through forgoing "the last 10 percent" and transferring them to other efforts to enhance health or safety. The local EPA administrator will be more likely to stop short of the last 10 percent in ordering cleanup of a New Hampshire site if he or she knows that some of the $9 million saved will actually be spent to help resolve other health problems instead of simply remaining in private pockets. One immediately thinks of a system that would encourage a settlement for, say, 50 percent, or even 25 percent, of the $9 million, and then transfer the settlement money to another project.[59] Still, the details of even such obvious "capture and transfer" projects may be difficult to work out, and transferring funds among different programs might prove yet more difficult. A deliberate, multi-program effort to create and implement such systems would make it more likely that the New Hampshire administrator will in fact stop short of that "last 10 percent."

The relation of the centralized administrative group to the problems of random agenda-setting and inconsistency is more obvious. The group's access to a broad range of different programs makes it more likely that less well-known programs (such as transportation for cancer checkups, or perhaps even efforts to stop the deforestation of Madagascar) will appear on agendas along with more traditional risk reduction. The group's agenda and system-building activities should help to produce uniform methods for measuring risks to humans that vary appreciably with scientific knowledge and circumstances. The group should begin to develop methods for measuring the effectiveness of similar programs in similar ways. One should expect to see the development of methods for examining the effect of one program's regulations upon another, and for inhibiting regulations that are shown to be counterproductive. More important, the group, after noticing that a little extra money spent on, say, vitamin supplements for pregnant women, or fireproofing space heaters would buy much more health safety than extra money spent on avoiding low-level radiation risks, would then ask what we should do about it. And, more generally, a politically insulated group could work with a sufficiently long time horizon to allow comprehensive regulation of risk, rather than responding in an extreme fashion to the latest health risk to catch public attention.[60]

4. *It is politically unacceptable.* The centralization of authority that the proposal embodies will tend to weaken the ability of Congressional subcommittees (or influential agency/outside-group/subcommittee "triangles")[61] to influence specific agency policies directly. Without some compensating degree of "group" independence from direct Presidential control, the proposal may not prove acceptable to many in the environmental community. But since many risk-related choices are, and must remain, inherently political, to insulate totally the group's major policy decisions from those of politically responsible officials is neither desirable nor possible.

Some degree of insulation can, however, be achieved, for example through the use of civil service career paths, by the professional discipline of staff members, by limiting the extent to which politically elected officials become involved in decisions about individual substances, and, if the public begins to recognize the group as a success, by a natural tendency for politicians to rely upon the group's decision as offering a partial refuge from responsibility for unpopular choices.

Nonetheless, you might still ask whether the group's work is sufficiently visible to the public—whether the group is sufficiently open to public participation to obtain the public's confidence. To some extent, of course, the group's proposals, plans, and findings would be openly available for comment and criticism. Yet one important objective is to limit the extent to which public debate about a particular substance determines the regulatory outcome, in respect to a range of substances that are not automatically or inevitably politically volatile. Is such an objective itself consistent with the building of public trust?

Remember the sharp decline in confidence in public institutions over the past twenty-five years. Recall, however, that rebuilt trust in institutions is based not simply on the public's perception of openness, but also on the ability of an institution to accomplish its mission successfully, particularly where that mission itself helps to achieve an important public purpose. Those who rebuilt confidence in the Federal Trade Commission in the 1970s did so not through public-relations campaigns but by reorganizing the Commission so that it better accomplished its important consumer-protection mission.[62] Doing so created better morale, increased confidence, and greater prestige, all of which improved the agency's reputation and in turn helped further improve agency performance. The Harris poll of confidence in public institutions presented earlier in this chapter offers some support for this view, for the institution that maintains the confidence of most Americans is the Armed Forces—not an open institution, but one which has successfully carried out its mission. Perhaps the Conseil d'Etat enjoys prestige in France for similar reasons. As I have said, France is not America; but a public that has become increasingly convinced that American politics resemble those of Fourth Republic France may find a corresponding need for, or virtue in, the Fourth Republic's civil service.

5. *There is no practical transition.* My proposal projects a small, powerful group of especially well-qualified civil servants. What cur-

rently exists is a more specialized, individual-agency-oriented civil service, traditionally controlled by two or three levels of non–civil service, transient political appointees. How do we get there from here?

The reason I believe that the proposal is practical is that it can begin with small changes. Unlike many proposals for change, which one must accept or reject wholesale, the suggestions made here can be implemented in small steps, permitting experiment at very little cost. To change the structure of OIRA, for example, by introducing more health and scientific personnel, charging the agency with finding methods to spend risk-regulation resources more effectively, and establishing a rotating career path, would not seem inordinately difficult. If the changes began to work, the organization would naturally begin to develop the added prestige and authority that would encourage future change.

Those who doubt this is possible should read the history of agency reform, for example, the reform of the Federal Trade Commission in the 1970s. FTC reformers initially brought about a few changes in personnel and organization, which were followed by small substantive successes in carrying out the agency's consumer-protection mandate, which in turn led to enhanced agency prestige, followed by Congressional willingness to delegate greater statutory authority, which permitted yet greater substantive success, all of which made it easier to attract better personnel. The self-reinforcing nature of each of these changes permitted the agency, rather like a snowball rolling downhill, to grow in effectiveness, prestige, and authority. The example suggests that substantive success (better substantive results) can breed power, which in turn (if used wisely) can yield yet more substantive success.

Even if the initial changes do not lead to such success, little would be lost. In light of the magnitude of the problems to which I have pointed, we might listen to FDR's advice that it "is common sense to take a method and try it. If it fails, admit it frankly and try another. But above all, try something."[63]

I shall conclude my discussion here, not simply because of lack of time or space or inclination, but because my suggestion, in its strongest form, would involve restructuring a central part of the Executive Branch. Reshaping an old institutional unit, or building a new one, involves more than simply trying to answer the problems of risk regulation. Other areas of governmental activity might also benefit from increased coordination and rationalization. One can find other important grounds, other arguments, supporting the need for this kind of structural change. (For example, the judicial tendency to review less closely than in the past agency policy determinations for reasonableness argues for some such centralized reviewing capacity,[64] perhaps within the Executive Branch itself. The courts' tendency, when interpreting statutes, to use legislative history less frequently and to rely more upon "canons of interpretation" argues for centralizing the drafting of statutes in the Executive Branch to help secure uniform judicial interpretations.)[65] The detailed form of any resulting institutional change would have to reflect such other needs and other arguments. Indeed, this book does claim to present the problem of risk regulation and its solution, but rather offers risk regulation as one substantive argument for greater centralized authority within the Executive Branch of government. This argument, one among several, shows a particular need, in an era of political fragmentation, for a reborn civil service.

Concluding Thoughts

In this book I have focused upon one kind of regulatory problem, the problem of regulating health risks. Yet it seems possible to satisfy Oliver Wendell Holmes's admonition to find general lessons in that particular. Let me suggest a few.

An examination of the problems of risk regulation offers a powerful counter-argument to the view that deregulation can solve all, or many, current problems of government regulation. It offers an equally strong counter-argument to the hopeful position that more direct "democratic" public involvement will automatically lead to better results (defining "better" nontautologically as results that the public itself wants). Such an examination suggests that the traditional New Deal notion of delegating broad, general legal authority to administrative bodies still retains its vitality.

My analysis of the problems surrounding risk regulation offers an important substantive argument against a "Balkanized" Executive Branch and suggests a need, extending beyond the subject itself, for more centralized coordination. It suggests the desirability of recruiting "coordinators" who are familiar with more than one discipline (not simply science, or law, or economics, or politics, or administration), more than one agency program, and more than one branch of government. It underscores the wisdom of Salvador DeMadriaga's aphorism, "He who is 'nothing but' is 'not even.'" Such cross-branch governmental experience does not teach any basic truths about government (other than clichés); but, in the context of a particular problem (say, risk regulation) it helps create solutions that reflect an understanding of and sensitivity to the likely reactions, the points of view, and the difficulties of those institutions, including those of that ultimate source of democratic legitimacy (which Congress very well reflects), the people.

Finally, this book also reflects a belief that trust in institutions arises not simply as a result of openness in government, responses to local interest groups, or priorities emphasized in the press—though these attitudes and actions play an important role—but also from those institutions' doing a difficult job well. A Socratic notion of virtue—the teachers teaching well, the students learning well, the judges judging well, and the health regulators more effectively bringing about better health—must be central in any effort to create the politics of trust.

NOTES

1. Systematic Problems

1. Cf. Henry Fairlie, "Fear of Living," *New Republic,* January 23, 1989, at 19 (inveighing against Americans' fear of everyday risks in everyday life).
2. Robert Cameron Mitchell and Richard T. Carson, "Valuing Drinking Water Reductions Using the Contingent Valuation Method: A Methodological Study of Risks from THM and Giardia" (1986) (Report prepared for the Office of Policy Analysis, United States Environmental Protection Agency, by Resources for the Future, Washington, D.C.). Mitchell developed this ladder to use in an exploratory survey he conducted in a small community in southern Illinois. The goal of the study was to measure the dollar values people were willing to pay for small reductions in the risk of dying from trihalomethanes in their drinking water. The risk levels are based on data in the literature available in 1985.
3. See 2A *Vital Statistics of the United States* 1 (1988) (table showing general mortality).
4. See *1987 Annual Cancer Statistics Review* I.20 (483,000 cancer deaths for all sites in 1987); American Cancer Society, *Cancer Facts and Figures—1992* 9 (520,000 cancer deaths estimated for 1992); Cristine Russell, "What, Me Worry?" *American Health,* June 1990, 45, 49; see also 2A *Vital Statistics of the United States* 11 (1988) (rate of 197.3 per 100,000 for all malignant neoplasms).
5. Richard Doll and Richard Peto, *The Causes of Cancer* 1256 (1981) (Table 20). See also Michael Gough, "Estimating Risks and Ignoring Killers," paper prepared for Cato Institute conference "Making Sense of Safety," March 21–22, 1991, at 4 ("Since the appearance of the Doll and Peto study, its findings have become widely accepted as the best approximation of cancer risks").
6. Doll and Peto, *The Causes of Cancer* 1256 (Table 20). See also Michael Gough, "Estimating Cancer Mortality: Epidemiological and Toxicological Methods Produce Similar Assessments," 23 *Envtl. Sci. & Tech.* 925 (1989) (finding that EPA's estimates, in *Unfinished Business* [1987], largely agreed with Doll and Peto's figure). But see Stephen Havas and Bailus Walker, Jr., "Massachusetts' Approach to the Prevention of Heart Disease, Cancer, and Stroke," 101 *U.S. Dep't of Health*

and Human Services Pub. Health Reps. 29 (1986) (giving a range of 10–20 percent for cancers attributable to occupational toxic exposures and 5–10 percent for environmental toxic exposures).

7. Michael Gough, at Resources for the Future, suggests that fully effective EPA regulation would reduce cancer deaths by between 1200 and 6600 each year. Michael Gough, "How Much Cancer Can EPA Regulate Away?" 10 *Risk Analysis* 1, 5 (1990). As Gough has noted elsewhere, "The lower estimate is 0.25 percent of the total of 485,000 annual cancer deaths, and the higher estimate is about 1.25 percent." Michael Gough, "Estimating Risks and Ignoring Killers," paper prepared for Cato Institute conference "Making Sense of Safety," March 21–22, 1991, at 7 (citing Gough, "How Much Cancer Can EPA Regulate Away?"). But see Philip J. Landrigan, "Commentary: Environmental Disease—A Preventable Epidemic," 82 *Am. J. Public Heath* 941 (1992) (suggesting that toxic diseases caused by work environment alone result in an estimated 50,000 to 70,000 deaths per year).

8. Doll and Peto, *The Causes of Cancer* 1256 (giving 30 percent as "best estimate" for proportion of cancer deaths attributable to tobacco, with a range of 25–40 percent); Stephen Havas and Bailus Walker, Jr., "Massachusetts' Approach to the Prevention of Heart Disease, Cancer, and Stroke," 101 *U.S. Department of Health and Human Services Pub. Health Reps.* 29 (1986) (30 percent).

9. See American Cancer Society, *Cancer Facts and Figures—1992* 3 (chart showing cancer death rates by site, indicating most cancers fairly constant, with rise in lung cancer and decline in stomach cancer and uterine cancer); Doll and Peto, *The Causes of Cancer,* at 1281–92; Eliot Marshall, "Experts Clash over Cancer Data," 250 *Science* 900, 902 (Nov. 16, 1990) (chart from U.S. Department of Health and Human Services showing most cancers in U.S. males fairly constant, with sharp rise in lung cancer and decline in stomach cancer); see also Richard Doll, "Are We Winning the Fight against Cancer? An Epidemiological Assessment," 26 *Eur. J. Cancer* 500 (1990) (answering yes); Richard D. Pollak, "The Science of Cancer," 106 *Public Interest* 122, 123 (Winter 1992) ("once the numbers are adjusted for age and population size, and if the special case of lung cancer is put aside, we see that cancer rates have not increased, and that for many cancers the rate of incidence is actually lower"). Cf. David G. Hoel, Devra L. Davis, Anthony B. Miller, Edward J. Sondik, and Anthony J. Swerdlow, "Trends in Cancer Mortality in 15 Industrialized Countries, 1969–1986," 84 *J. Nat'l Cancer Inst.* 313 (1992) (noting rises in incidence of some cancers). But see Devra Lee Davis, David Hoel, John Fox, and Alan Lopez, "International Trends in Cancer Mortality in France, West Germany, Italy, Japan, England and Wales, and the USA," 336 *Lancet* 474 (Aug. 25, 1990) (observing increased incidence of all cancers other than lung and stomach—that is, brain and other central nervous system cancer, breast cancer, multiple myeloma, kidney cancer, non-Hodgkin lymphoma, and melanoma—in persons aged 55 and over); John C. Bailar, "Death from All Cancers: Trends in Sixteen Countries," 609 *Annals N.Y.*

Acad. Sci. 49 (1990) (rates rising, especially among older age groups); Samuel S. Epstein, "Losing the War against Cancer: Who's to Blame and What to Do about It," 20 *International J. Health Services* 53 (1990). Cf. Catherine Hall, Ellen Benhamou, and Françoise Doyon, "Trends in Cancer Mortality," 336 *Lancet* 1262 (Nov. 17, 1990) (letter to editor) (criticizing *Lancet* paper by Davis et al., *supra*); Stan C. Freni, "Trends in Cancer Mortality," 336 *Lancet* 1263 (Nov. 17, 1990) (letter to editor) (same); André E. M. McLean, "International Trends in Cancer Mortality," 336 *Lancet* 816 (Sept. 29, 1990) (letter to editor) (same); Devra Lee Davis, David Hoel, John Fox, and Alan Lopez, "Trends in Cancer Morality," 336 *Lancet* 1265 (Nov. 17, 1990) (letter to editor) (responding to criticisms). See generally Marshall, "Experts Clash over Cancer Data," (discussing debate concerning cancer rates); Devra Lee Davis and David G. Hoel, "International Trends in Cancer Mortality," 6(2) *Health & Environment Digest* 1 (May 1992) (discussing data suggesting increase in cancer rates).

10. American Cancer Society, *Cancer Facts and Figures—1992* 3 (chart).

11. See Federal Focus, Inc., *Toward Common Measures: Recommendations for a Presidential Executive Order in Environmental Risk Assessment and Risk Management Policy* 20–23 (1991) (listing principal environmental health and safety statutes and responsible agencies); see also Lave and Upton, *Toxic Chemicals, Waste and the Environment* 29 (1988) (listing thirteen more widely used statutes: FDCA, FFRA, CAA, OSHA, CPSA, FWPCA, FEPCA, SDWA, TSCA, RICRA, HMTA, CERCLA, and SARA).

12. Comprehensive Environmental Response, Compensation, and Liability Act of 1980, 42 U.S.C. §§9601 et seq.

13. Toxic Substances Control Act, 15 U.S.C. §§2601 et seq.

14. Federal Insecticide, Fungicide, and Rodenticide Act, 7 U.S.C. §§121 et seq.

15. Clean Air Act, 42 U.S.C. §§7401 et seq.

16. Occupational Safety and Health Act of 1970, 29 U.S.C. §§651 et seq.

17. Food, Drug, and Cosmetic Act of 1938, 21 U.S.C. §§301 et seq.

18. Atomic Energy Act of 1954, 42 U.S.C. §§2011 et seq.

19. Committee on the Institutional Means for Assessment of Risks to Public Health, *Risk Assessment in the Federal Government: Managing the Process* 18-19 (1983).

20. See id. at 18-33; Milton Russell and Michael Gruber, "Risk Assessment in Environmental Policy-Making," 236 *Science* 286 (April 17, 1987) ("Risk assessment at EPA proceeds in four steps: (i) hazard assessment, (ii) dose-response assessment, (iii) exposure assessment, and (iv) risk characterization"); see generally John J. Cohrssen and Vincent T. Covello, *Risk Analysis: A Guide to Principles and Methods for Analyzing Health and Environmental Risks* (1989) (explaining in detail stages of risk assessment); Lester B. Lave, "Methods of Risk Assessment," in *Quantitative Risk Assessment in Regulation* 23 (Lave, ed., 1982).

21. George C. Pimentel, "Let's Talk about Chemistry," *The Chemist,* November

1987, at 6 (quoted in Carl B. Meyer, "The Environmental Fate of Toxic Waters, the Certainty of Harm, Toxic Torts, and Toxic Regulation," 19 *Envtl. L.* 321, 327 n.20 [1988]).

22. See W. Kip Viscusi, "Toward a Diminished Role for Tort Liability: Social Insurance, Government Regulation, and Contemporary Risks to Health and Safety," 6 *Yale J. on Reg.* 65, 92–93 (1989).

23. The former Superfund project manager Leo Levenson, "Unnecessary Risks," Graduate School of Public Policy, University of California, Berkeley (Dec. 6, 1989), quoted in Aaron Wildavsky, "If Claims of Harm from Technology Are False, Mostly False, or Unproven, What Does That Tell Us about Science?" in *Health, Lifestyle, and Environment: Countering the Panic* at 111, 115 n. 9 (Social Affairs Unit, Manhattan Institute, 1991).

24. See generally National Research Council, *Environmental Epidemiology: Public Health and Hazardous Wastes* (1991) (surveying weaknesses in Superfund approach and lack of attention to actual risks).

25. A recent study found that about 90 percent of insurers' and 20 percent of liable firms' expenditure on Superfund environmental claims was not on actual cleanup but instead on "transaction costs," the bulk of which was legal fees. Enforcement costs accounted for 11 percent of EPA's Superfund expenditure, with an unknown percentage spent on transaction costs. Jan Paul Acton and Lloyd S. Dixon, *Superfund and Transaction Costs: The Experiences of Insurers and Very Large Industrial Firms* xi, xiii, xv (RAND Corporation, Institute for Civil Justice, 1992). See also John C. Butler III, "Superfund: Super Costs," *Rethinking Superfund: It Costs Too Much; It's Unfair; It Must Be Fixed* 67 (National Legal Center for the Public Interest, 1991) (discussing causes of high transaction costs, and suggesting [at 68] that overall, 10–15 percent of direct cleanup costs, or about $4 million average per National Priority List site, may be a conservative estimate of transaction costs).

26. See Sheldon Meyers, "Applications of De Minimis," in *De Minimis Risk* 102 (Chris Whipple, ed., 1987) (discussing the importance of the use of "de minimis" considerations in risk analysis where "it frequently is relatively cheap to reduce risks from 0 to 90 percent, more expensive to go from 90 percent to 99 percent, and more expensive to go from 99 percent to 99.9 percent").

27. *United States v. Ottati & Goss, Inc.,* 900 F.2d 429 (1st Cir. 1990).

28. See id., 900 F.2d at 431–32, 436, 440–41. The specific chemicals involved are listed in the district court's opinion concerning liability, *United States v. Ottati & Goss, Inc.,* 630 F. Supp. 1361, 1383–90 (D.N.H. 1985). See also Gloria J. Hathaway, Nick H. Proctor, James P. Hughes, and Michael L. Fischman, *Proctor and Hughes' Chemical Hazards of the Workplace* (3d ed. 1991) (providing information on chemicals listed in *Ottati & Goss*).

29. *Ottati & Goss,* 900 F.2d at 436, 441.

30. See *Ottati & Goss,* 630 F. Supp. at 1366.

31. *Ottati & Goss,* 900 F.2d at 441.

32. *Ottati & Goss,* 900 F.2d at 440.

33. See "Asbestos," *Mining Magazine* (November 1989), at 411 (95 percent of world production is chrysotile, or white, asbestos; amphibole asbestos includes crocidolite [blue] and amosite [brown] asbestos).

34. See B. T. Mossman, J. Bignon, M. Corn, A. Seaton, and J. B. L. Gee, "Asbestos: Scientific Developments and Implications for Public Policy," 247 *Science* 294, 299 (Jan. 19, 1990); Health Effects Institute—Asbestos Research, *Asbestos in Public and Commercial Buildings: A Literature Review and Synthesis of Current Knowledge* 1–9 (1991); Devra Lee Davis and Barbara Mandula, "Airborne Asbestos and Public Health," 6 *Ann. Rev. Public Health* 195 (1985); see also Bernard Gee, "Asbestos: Better Off Left Alone," *Toronto Star,* Dec. 4, 1990, at A21.

35. Health Effects Institute—Asbestos Research, *Asbestos in Public and Commercial Buildings: A Literature Review and Synthesis of Current Knowledge* 1-10 to 1-11 (1991) (Table 1-1). For a sample of the kinds of disagreement among scientists over, for example, just how dangerous white asbestos fibers may be, see, e.g., Arnold R. Brody, "Asbestos, Carcinogenicity, and Public Policy," 248 *Science* 795 (May 18, 1990) (letter to the editor) ("I am not convinced that it is prudent to consider chrysotile asbestos fibers innocuous"); William J. Nicholson, Edward M. Johnson, John S. Harington, James Melius, and Philip J. Landrigan, "Asbestos, Carcinogenicity, and Public Policy," 248 *Science* 796 (May 18, 1990) (letter to the editor) (arguing that evidence shows danger from chrysotile fibers); B. T. Mossman, J. Bignon, M. Corn, A. Seaton, and J. B. L. Gee, "Asbestos, Carcinogenicity, and Public Policy," 248 *Science* 799 (May 18, 1990) (letter to the editor) (responding to letters); Wilson da Silva, "Study Shows Tripling of Asbestos Fatalities in Decade," *Reuter Library Report,* February 27, 1991 (discussing National Institute of Occupational Health and Safety study) ("The study also shows that white asbestos, formerly suspected of being benign, also produces cancer. Previously blue asbestos was believed to be the main cause of mesothelioma"). Cf. Richard Stone, "No Meeting of the Minds on Asbestos," 254 *Science* 928 (Nov. 15, 1991) (discussing divide among experts on dangers of chrysotile [white] asbestos).

36. B. T. Mossman, J. Bignon, M. Corn, A. Seaton, and J. B. L. Gee, "Asbestos: Scientific Developments and Implications for Public Policy," 247 *Science* 294, 299 (Jan. 19, 1990).

37. Id. at 299 (Table 2) (showing annual rate of 0.005 to 0.093 deaths per million students exposed for five years). Cf. Kenny S. Crump, "Asbestos, Carcinogenicity, and Public Policy," 248 *Science* 799 (May 18, 1990) (letter to the editor) (providing small correction to figures in table of Mossman et al.); B. T. Mossman, J. Bignon, M. Corn, A. Seaton, J. B. L. Gee, "Asbestos, Carcinogenicity, and Public Policy," 248 *Science* 799, 801 (May 18, 1990) (letter to the editor) (acknowledging Crump's correction).

38. Mossman et al., *supra* note 36, at 299. See also Jay Mathews, "To Yank or Not to Yank?" *Newsweek,* April 13, 1992, at 59 (discussing controversy about abatement).

39. Mossman et al., *supra* note 36, at 294.

40. Calculations assume 13 million new cars per year. The figure of 50,000 auto deaths per year is high: the National Safety Council put the total for 1991 at 43,500. Source: American Automobile Manufacturers' Association, telephone interview.

41. Kelly Richmond, "Bryan's Airbag Proposal Added to Highway Bill," *States News Service*, June 12, 1991 (airbags cost $200 per car); Andrea Neal, "Court Refuses to Intervene in Air Bag Case," *UPI*, March 30, 1987 ($320 per car, and over $800 to replace; airbags estimated to save between 3,780 and 9,110 lives per year); see also Lester B. Lave, "Conflicting Objectives in Regulating the Automobile," 212 *Science* 893, 895 (May 22, 1981) ($300 to $580 cost per car for airbags, with a cost per life saved of $1.03–2 million).

42. *Corrosion Proof Fittings v. E.P.A.*, 947 F.2d 1201 (5th Cir. 1991).

43. The EPA's regulation was promulgated at 54 Fed. Reg. 29459 (1989), to be codified at 40 C.F.R. 763.

44. See 947 F.2d at 1219, 1222, 1226.

45. 947 F.2d at 1222.

46. Id.

47. Id.

48. 947 F.2d at 1223.

49. *Corrosion Proof Fittings*, 947 F.2d at 1223 n.23 (citing Lawrence D. Budnick, "Toothpick-Related Injuries in the United States, 1979 through 1982," 252 *JAMA* 796 [Aug. 10, 1984]). But see also Lester B. Lave, "Health and Safety Risk Analyses: Information for Better Decisions," in 236 *Science* 291, 293 (Apr. 17, 1987) ("Is having brightly colored maraschino cherries worth even a minuscule threat [the risk of red food color is estimated to be 0.02 cancer(s) per million lifetimes]?") (citations omitted).

50. See 29 U.S.C. §655.

51. 43 Fed. Reg. 5918–70 (1978).

52. *See Industrial Union Dept., AFL-CIO v. American Petroleum Inst.*, 448 U.S. 607, 631–38 (1980) (Opinion of Stevens, J.).

53. Id.; see generally John D. Graham, Laura C. Green, and Marc J. Roberts, *In Search of Safety: Chemicals and Cancer Risk* 80–88 (1988) (discussing the making of the first OSHA rules on benzene and the Supreme Court decision).

54. See Graham, Green, and Roberts, *In Search of Safety*, at 88–91.

55. See 52 Fed. Reg. 34462–63, 34493–504 (1987).

56. M. Aksoy, S. Erdem, and G. Dincol, "Types of Leukemia in Chronic Benzene Poisoning," 55 *Acta Haematologica* 65 (1976).

57. E. C. Vigliani and G. Saita, "Benzene and Leukemia," 271 *New Eng. J. Med.* 872 (1964).

58. R. A. Rinksy, R. J. Young, and A. B. Smith, "Leukemia in Benzene Workers," 2 *Am. J. Indus. Med.* 217 (1981).

59. M. G. Ott, J. C. Townsend, W. A. Fishbeck, and R. A. Langner, "Mortality among Individuals Occupationally Exposed to Benzene," 33 *Archives of Environmental Health* 3 (1978).

60. See 52 Fed. Reg. 34492–501; see also Hathaway, Proctor, Hughes, and Fischman, *Chemical Hazards of the Workplace,* at 103–05 (discussing benzene studies); Graham, Green, and Roberts, *In Search of Safety,* at 115-50 (discussing studies concerning benzene and leukemia).

61. This is a question of considerable scientific debate. See, e.g., Mary C. White, Peter F. Infante, and Kenneth C. Chu, "A Quantitative Estimate of Leukemia Mortality Associated with Occupational Exposure to Benzene," 2 *Risk Analysis* 195 (1982); Jerry L. R. Chandler, "Benzene and the One-Hit Model," 4 *Risk Analysis* 7 (1984); Harland Austin, Elizabeth Delzell, and Philip Cole, "Benzene and Leukemia: A Review of the Literature and a Risk Assessment," 127 *Am. J. Epidemiology* 419 (1988).

62. See 52 Fed. Reg. 34462–63, 34490–91. The 1987 final rule has not been challenged, according to a telephone interview with Melodie Sands, Occupational Safety and Health Administration, March 31, 1992.

63. See 52 Fed. Reg. 34461.

64. 42 U.S.C. §7412(d).

65. See National Emission Standards for Hazardous Air Pollutants; Benzene Emissions from Chemical Manufacturing Process Vents, Industrial Solvent Use, Benzene Waste Operations, Benzene Transfer Operations, and Gasoline Marketing System, 55 Fed. Reg. 8292 (1990); National Emission Standards for Hazardous Air Pollutants; Benzene Emissions from Maleic Anhydride Plants, Ethylbenzene/Styrene Plants, Benzene Storage Vessels, Benzene Equipment Leaks, and Coke By-Product Recovery Plants, 54 Fed. Reg. 38044 (1989). EPA, like OSHA, assumed a linear dose/response relationship. See 55 Fed. Reg. 8305; 54 Fed. Reg. 38063. EPA's approach to benzene was guided by the decision of the United States Court of Appeals for the District of Columbia in *Natural Resources Defense Council v. U.S. E.P.A.,* 824 F.2d 1146 (1987), in which the court construed section 112(d) of the Clean Air Act, which requires EPA to set emission standards "at the level which . . . provides an ample margin of safety to the public health." Id. at 1147 (quoting former version of 42 U.S.C. §7412(b)(1)(B)). This provision of the Clean Air Act was modified by the 1990 amendments (see 42 U.S.C. §7412, current version), which are in turn critiqued in Janet L. McQuaid, "Risk Assessment of Hazardous Air Pollutants under the EPA's Final Benzene Rules and the Clean Air Act Amendments of 1990," 70 *Tex. L. Rev.* 427 (1991); and Nichols, "Comparing Risk Standards," 90–92.

66. See Nichols, "Comparing Risk Standards," 92 (Table 1); see also 55 Fed. Reg. 8294, 9298; 54 Fed. Reg. 38050, 38051, 38054.

67. For a thorough discussion of arguments about human life valuation and cost-effectiveness methodology generally, see W. Kip Viscusi, *Risk by Choice: Regulating Health Safety in the Workplace* 22–52 (1983).

68. Paul Slovic, "Perception of Risk," 236 *Science* 280, 283–84 (April 17, 1987).

69. *In re Agent Orange Product Liability Litigation,* 597 F. Supp. 740, 857 (E.D.N.Y. 1984).

70. *In re Agent Orange Product Liability Litigation,* 611 F. Supp. 1233, 1260 (E.D.N.Y. 1985).

71. See, e.g., Science Panel of the Cabinet Council Agent Orange Working Group, "The State of Agent Orange Related Research in the Federal Government" 2 (1985) ("Based on the growing body of information in hand, the worst case scenarios envisioned by some as a consequence of exposure to [Agent Orange] are not being realized. Populations known or possibly exposed to [Agent Orange] which are being studied have not so far exhibited increased incidence of cancer, or death from other causes, or abnormally high rates of birth defects in their offspring. This optimism is tempered by knowledge that other, less-well characterized effects of concern may be associated with [Agent Orange]"); Press Release, "Air Force Releases Ranch Hand Baseline Morbidity Study" (February 24, 1984); Lawrence B. Hobson, "Epidemiology of Soft-Tissue Sarcoma and Related Human Research (As Related to Herbicide Exposure)" 15 (Veterans Administration, March 1983) ("At best, the Scottish verdict of 'not proven' seems most realistic at this time . . . 'there is still no evidence that [herbicides or dioxin contaminants in Agent Orange] are mutagenic, carcinogenic, or teratogenic in man, nor that they have caused reproductive difficulties in the human'"), quoting Council on Scientific Affairs' Advisory Panel on Toxic Substances (American Medical Association), "The Health Effects of 'Agent Orange' and Polychlorinated Dioxin Contaminants," (October 1, 1981); Air Force Health Study (with Science Applications Int'l Corporation), "An Epidemiologic Investigation of Health Effects in Air Force Personnel Following Exposure to Herbicides," Abstract (March 1991) (dioxin found to have significant associations with diabetes, percent body fat [and related conditions], cholesterol, HDL and cholesterol-HDL ratio but not with other health variables); R. R. Suskind and V. S. Hertzberg, "Human Health Effects of 2,4,5-T and Its Toxic Contaminants," 251 *JAMA* 2372 (May 11, 1984) (exposure linked to chloracne and gastrointestinal tract ulcers but not to cardiovascular disease, hepatic disease, renal damage, or nervous system problems); A. L. Young, M. R. Flicker, H. K. Kang, and B. M. Shepard, "Health Surveillance of Vietnam Veterans Claiming Agent Orange Exposure" 17 (Veterans Administration, 1984) (Agent Orange registry, despite limitations, can still "serve a useful purpose in suggesting areas for further in-depth review and study").

72. Bruce N. Ames, Renae Magaw, and Lois Swirsky Gold, "Ranking Possible Carcinogenic Hazards," 236 *Science* 271, 273 (Table 1) (April 17, 1987). Recent evidence suggests that more heavily chlorinated PCBs may be far more carcinogenic than less heavily chlorinated PCBs. Hence, broad prohibitions on all PCBs may be inappropriate. See the letter from John A. Moore, President, Institute for Evaluating Health Risks, to Hank Habicht, Deputy Administrator, Environmental Protection Agency (July 1, 1991), in Institute for Evaluating Health Risks, *Reassessment of Liver Findings in Five PCB Studies in Rats* (1991).

73. See Bruce N. Ames, Renae Magaw, and Lois Swirsky Gold, "Ranking Possible Carcinogenic Hazards," 236 *Science* 271, 273 (Table 1) (April 17, 1987).

74. See Bruce N. Ames, Renae Magaw, and Lois Swirsky Gold, "Ranking Possible Carcinogenic Hazards," 236 *Science* 271, 277 (April 17, 1987) ("The aflatoxin in the average peanut butter sandwich, or a raw mushroom, are 75 and 200 times, respectively, the possible hazard of EDB"); Richard B. Belzer, "The Peril and Promise of Risk Assessment," 14(4) *Regulation* 40, 48 (Fall 1991) (same); Lester B. Lave, "Health and Safety Risk Analyses: Information for Better Decisions," 236 *Science* 291, 293 (April 17, 1987) ("The tolerance level of aflatoxin in corn is estimated to increase the incidence of cancer by as much as 700 per million lifetimes") (citations omitted); Richard Wilson, "Summary and Analysis," in 16 *Envtl. L. Rep.* 10226 (August 1986) (aflatoxin in peanut butter [at 20 parts per billion] is a thousand times more carcinogenic than EDB, banned at the same level); Harold Issadore Sharlin, "Macro-Risks, Micro-Risks, and the Media: The EDB Case," in *The Social and Cultural Construction of Risk* 183 (B. B. Johnson and V. T. Covello, eds., 1987) (suggesting that EPA failed to inform public adequately concerning actual risks). For a sympathetic account of EPA's regulation of EDB, suggesting that the agency appropriately "partitioned risk," see Milton Russell and Michael Gruber, "Risk Assessment in Environmental Policy-Making," 236 *Science* 286, 288 (April 17, 1987).

75. *Regulatory Program of the United States Government, April 1, 1991–March 31, 1992,* at 12, table 2 (listing cost-effectiveness of hazardous waste land disposal ban rule for "first third" as $4.19 billion per premature death averted).

76. Troyce Jones, "Radiological and Chemical Contamination: Should I Spend Money for the Present or the Future?" 15(5) *Health Physics Soc'y Newsl.* 1–4 (1987).

77. Milton Russell and Michael Gruber, "Risk Assessment in Environmental Policy-Making," 236 *Science* 286, 288 (April 17, 1987).

78. See *supra* note 7.

79. See *supra* note 25.

80. Risk regulation seems to be the major focus of current governmental regulatory efforts. See Stephen G. Breyer and Richard B. Stewart, *Administrative Law and Regulatory Policy* 165–66 (3d ed., 1992).

81. Peter Passell, "Experts Question Staggering Costs of Toxic Cleanups," *N.Y. Times,* Sept. 1, 1991, at A1, A28.

82. Milton Russell, E. William Colglazier, and Mary English, *Hazardous Waste Remediation: The Task Ahead* (Waste Management Research and Education Institute, University of Tennessee, Dec. 10, 1991), 16.

83. See Carnegie Commission on Science, Technology, and Government, E^3: *Organizing for Environment, Energy, and the Economy in the Executive Branch of the U.S. Government* 5 n.3 (April 1990), citing C. A. Zraket, "Opening Remarks—Environmental Situation in the United States," in A. T. Amr, D. E. Egan, K. R. Krickenberger, and S. V. McBrien, "Pollution Prevention: Oppor-

tunities and Constraints" at 3 (Workshop Presentations and Summary) (August 1989).

84. The Department of Energy has also estimated that, due to its failure to comply with Clean Water Act standards at federal sites, "taxpayers may pay $40 to $70 billion during the next 20 years to clean up or contain the contamination at its facilities." *United States Dep't of Energy v. Ohio,* 112 S. Ct. 1627, 1640–41 (1992) (White, J., concurring), citing "Cleanup at Federal Facilities: Hearing on H.R. 765 before the Subcommittee on Transportation and Hazardous Materials of the House Committee on Energy and Commerce," 101st Cong., 1st Sess., Ser. No. 101-4, p. 44 (1989).

85. See Federal Focus, Inc., *Toward Common Measures: Recommendations for a Presidential Executive Order in Environmental Risk Assessment and Risk Management Policy* 8 and n.2 (1991) (noting that compliance with pollution control laws has been estimated to cost between $100 and $115 billion per year) (listing sources). "According to the Department of Commerce, the nation spent about $78 billion in 1986 on all forms of environmental protection, about two-thirds in industry." Carnegie Commission on Science, Technology, and Government, E^3: *Organizing for Environment, Energy, and the Economy in the Executive Branch of the U.S. Government* 5 n.2 (April 1990), citing K. D. Farber and G. L. Rutledge, "Pollution Abatement and Control Expenditures, 1983–1986," in *Survey of Current Business* 28 (May 1988), and Congressional Office of Technology Assessment, "Serious Reduction of Hazardous Waste for Pollution Prevention and Industrial Efficiency," in OTA-ITE-317 (1986).

86. See *supra* note 28.

87. In 1990, EPA estimated average total cleanup costs for each of the (then) 1187 National Priorities List sites at $31.6 million (1988 dollars). EPA, National Priorities List for Uncontrolled Hazardous Waste Sites, 55 Fed. Reg. 35,502, 35,511 (Aug. 30, 1990), now codified and updated at 40 C. F. R. 300 (1992). By early 1992, the NPL had expanded to 1250 sites, and EPA was predicting an annual addition of 100 sites; and academic estimates of average (currently listed) site cleanup cost had reached $40 million (Resources for the Future) and $50 million (University of Tennessee). Katherine N. Probst and Paul R. Portney, *Assigning Liability for Superfund Cleanups* (Resources for the Future, 1992), at 51, 17, 30.

88. A report prepared for the EPA and recently released by the Senate Committee on Governmental Affairs indicates that there may be as many as 45,000 sites nationwide that are polluted with radioactive materials. See John H. Cushman, Jr., "Report Lists 45,000 Potential Radioactive Sites," *N.Y. Times,* Apr. 9, 1992, at A14.

89. The Federal Government has recently announced a program to immunize children under the age of two against preventable diseases. See Robert Pear, "Bush Announces New Effort to Immunize Children," *N.Y. Times,* May 12, 1992, at

A18. (But "pediatricians and other public health experts said [the] . . . proposal was belated and inadequate.")

90. Stephen L. Cochi, Claire V. Broome and Allen W. Hightower, "Immunization of US Children with Hemophilus Influenzae Type b Polysaccharide Vaccine: A Cost-Effectiveness Model of Strategy Assessment," 253 *JAMA* 521 (1985).

91. P. J. van der Maas et al., *The Costs and Effects of Mass Screening for Breast Cancer (De Kosten en Effecten van Bevolkingsonderzoek op Borstkanker)* 52 (Department of Public Health and Social Medicine, Erasmus Universiteit Rotterdam et al.) (trans. 1988). According to Margaret Maxey, "Breast cancer claims more than 32,000 actual lives each year. Yet the breast cancer research budget of the National Cancer Institute was only $81 million for 1990 and $90.2 million for 1991." Margaret N. Maxey, "Regulating Safety in the Name of Ethics: A Fatally Flawed Experiment?" paper prepared for Cato Institute conference "Making Sense of Safety," March 21–22, 1991, at 22. See also Jocelyn White, "Superfund: Pouring Money Down a Hole," *N.Y. Times,* April 17, 1992, at A27 (arguing that too much is spent on Superfund cleanups for too little and noting that "an estimated 175,900 breast cancer cases are diagnosed each year. The National Cancer Institute's 1993 budget for breast cancer research is $133 million"). Mammograms are not as dramatically cost effective—although they may still be helpful—in all age groups. Studies suggest that they are at their most effective for older women; indeed, for young women, who are at far less risk of actually having breast cancer, the increased risk of radiogenic cancer from the testing process itself may outweigh the benefits of the assay. See Elisabeth Rosenthal, "Study Revives Debate on Need for Mammograms before 50," *N.Y. Times,* May 13, 1992, at C12; Lester B. Lave, "Health and Safety Analyses: Information for Better Decisions," 236 *Science* 291, 292 (Apr. 17, 1987). See also David G. Hoel, Devra L. Davis, Anthony B. Miller, Edward J. Sondik, and Anthony J. Swerdlow, "Trends in Cancer Mortality in 15 Industrialized Countries, 1969–1986," *J. Nat'l Cancer Inst.* 313, 317 (1992) (table 3) (showing mortality rates for breast cancer rising from 45 per 100,000 among women 45–54 years old to 136 per 100,000 among those age 75–84); Sandra Blakeslee, "Faulty Math Heightens Fears of Breast Cancer," *N.Y. Times,* Mar. 15, 1992, at D1 (risk of breast cancer much higher among older women than younger women). Cf. Elizabeth Rosenthal, "Scientists Face Rumor on Cancer," *N.Y. Times,* May 5, 1992, at C11 (discussing Canadian study suggesting no benefit for certain age groups from routine mammograms).

92. Lester B. Lave, "Methods of Risk Assessment," in *Quantitative Risk Assessment Regulation* 23, 28 (Lave, ed., 1982).

93. See Lester B. Lave, "Viscusi's *Risk by Choice: Regulating Health and Safety in the Workplace,*" in 14 *Bell J. Econ.* 607, 609 (1983). Cf. Lester B. Lave, "An Economic Approach to Protecting Worker Health and Safety," 44 (12) *Am. Ind. Hyg. Assoc. J.* A-22 (1983) (discussing OSHA's failure to regulate workplace safety).

94. U.S. General Accounting Office, *Toxic Substances: EPA's Chemical Testing Program Has Made Little Progress* 13 (Government Printing Office, April 1990).

95. Id. at 2.

96. Id. at 21.

97. Id. at 21.

98. Id. at 24–25. For a suggested battery of short-term assays to help create an effective and efficient organization to EPA testing, see Lester B. Lave and Gilbert S. Omenn, "Cost-Effectiveness of Short-Term Tests for Carcinogenicity," 324 *Nature* 29 (Nov. 6, 1986).

99. See Lester B. Lave, "Does the Surgeon General Need a Statistics Advisor?" in *Chance: New Directions for Statistics and Computing* 33, 39 (1990) (rodent bioassays cost $1 million and take three years to perform); Lester B. Lave, Fanny K. Ennever, Herbert S. Rosenkranz, and Gilbert S. Omenn, "Information Value of the Rodent Bioassay," 336 *Nature* 631, 632 (Dec. 15, 1988), citing *Chemical and Engineering News* 24 (June 8, 1987).

100. Recently EPA has reported that the dangers of dioxin had been overstated. See Keith Schneider, "U.S. Officials Say Dangers of Dioxin Were Exaggerated," *N.Y. Times,* Aug. 15, 1991, at A1 ("The revised view of the dangers of dioxin has raised serious concerns within the E.P.A., which used many of the same procedures to determine the hazards of dioxin as it did to set air and water pollution limits for most of the other chemicals that the agency regulates. If . . . dioxin is much less dangerous than had been determined, that could mean the Government's regulations for other compounds will need to be adjusted"). See also Christine Gorman, "The Double Take on Dioxin," *Time* 52 (Aug. 26, 1991).

101. See U.S. Congress, Office of Technology Assessment, *Neurotoxicity: Identifying and Controlling Poisons of the Nervous System* (1990); Richard Stone, "Zeroing in on Brain Toxins," 255 *Science* 1063 (Feb. 28, 1992) (discussing report, "Environmental Neurotoxicity," published by National Research Council). See also Federal Focus, Inc., *Toward Common Measures: Recommendations for a Presidential Executive Order in Environmental Risk Assessment and Risk Management Policy* 67–69 (1991).

102. *Neurotoxicity, supra* note 101, at 304.

103. Id. at 304. See also Jon R. Luoma, "New Effect of Pollutants: Hormone Mayhem," *N.Y. Times,* Mar. 24, 1992, at C1 (describing deleterious effects of pollutants [e.g., DDT, dioxin, and PCBs] on hormonal systems of animals, in addition to their being carcinogenic).

104. U.S. Environmental Protection Agency, *Unfinished Business: A Comparative Assessment of Environmental Problems* (1987).

105. Science Advisory Board, U.S. Environmental Protection Agency, *Reducing Risk: Setting Priorities and Strategies for Environmental Protection* (1990). But see Senator David Durenberger, "A Dissenting Voice," *EPA Journal* (Mar./Apr. 1991) (criticizing EPA's conclusions in *Unfinished Business* and the

EPA SAB's in *Reducing Risk,* contending that efforts to prioritize health and environmental risks by means of comparative risk assessment may be fundamentally flawed).

106. See Leslie Roberts, "Counting On Science at EPA," 249 *Science* 616 (Aug. 10, 1990) (comparing public and experts' priorities); see also Paul Slovic, "Perception of Risk," 236 *Science* 280, 281 (April 17, 1987).

107. Michael Gough, "How Much Cancer Can EPA Regulate Away?" 10 *Risk Analysis* 1, 5 (1990).

108. *Regulatory Program of the United States Government, April 1, 1991– March 31, 1992* at 12 (Table 2).

109. Id.

110. See W. Kip Viscusi, "Toward a Diminished Role for Tort Liability: Social Insurance, Government Regulation, and Contemporary Risks to Health and Safety," 6 *Yale J. on Reg.* 65, 80–81 (1989) (collecting results of studies yielding estimates ranging from $676,000 to $12 million); Michael J. Moore and W. Kip Viscusi, "Doubling the Estimated Value of Life: Results Using the New Occupational Fatality Data," in 7 *J. Policy Analysis & Mgmt.* 476, 486 (1988) (discussing estimates of both $2 million, using data from the Bureau of Labor Statistics, and $5–6 million, using data from the National Institute of Occupational Safety's National Traumatic Occupational Fatality project); see also W. Kip Viscusi, *Fatal Tradeoffs: Public and Private Responsibilities for Risk* 263–65 (1992) (listing cost per life saved for various regulations compared to valuations of life saved).

111. On the general problem, see Richard B. Belzer, "The Peril and Promise of Risk Assessment," 14(4) *Regulation* 40, 47–48 (Fall 1991); OMB, *Regulatory Program of the United States Government, April 1, 1990–March 31, 1991* 24–25. For the sewage sludge example, see id. at 25; Richard B. Belzer, "Risk Assessment as a Tool for Decision Making: Is It Benign or Malignant?" paper presented at Cato Institute conference "Making Sense of Safety," March 1991, at 16. The proposed sewage sludge rule appears in U.S. Environmental Protection Agency, "Standards for the Disposal of Sewage Sludge: Proposed Rule," 54 Fed. Reg. 5746 (Feb. 6, 1989). According to Milton Russell and Michael Gruber, "Risk Assessment in Environmental Policy-Making," 236 *Science* 286, 289 (April 17, 1989), "the removal of pollutants from waste water produces sludge that must be either disposed of on land, incinerated, or dumped at sea. None of these procedures are without risk to human health or the environment." But see EPA, "Interagency Policy on Beneficial Use of Municipal Sludge on Federal Land," 56 Fed. Reg. 33,186, 33,188 (July 18, 1991) ("The weight of scientific evidence supports the presumption that beneficial use of sludge that is permitted by EPA or the States and is of such quality to ensure compliance with the permit does not present a significant risk to the environment when appropriately applied to the land").

112. For example, Massachusetts Water Resource Authority (MWRA) prohibits

discharge into its sewage system of more than 1 mg./liter of zinc. 360 CMR 10.024(2) (May 1, 1987, as amended). Asked to comment on suggestions that this might increase the costs associated with zinc ointment used with regular diapers and so induce people to substitute disposable diapers, leading to landfill problems, an official at MWRA responded that he was not aware of such cost implications; asked whether they might lead to increased use of disposable diapers, he replied, "I suppose so" (telephone interview, August 27, 1992). For doubts concerning the recyclability of disposable diapers, see, e.g., PR Newswire, "Washington Citizens for Recycling Foundation: Question of Disposable Diaper Recyclability Raised in Suit of Anderson," (June 29, 1992) (noting finding of the City of Seattle Solid Waste Utility in 1991 that recycling of disposable diapers is infeasible, and 1991 settlement between Procter & Gamble and the Attorneys General of ten states which prohibited use of the term "recyclable").

113. Richard B. Belzer, "The Peril and Promise of Risk Assessment," 14(4) *Regulation* 40, 48 (Fall 1991). Belzer notes that the EPA eventually retrieved its error by exempting CFCs from the hazardous waste regulation.

114. *Competitive Enterprise Inst. v. NHTSA*, 956 F.2d 321, 327 (D.C. Cir. 1992). For evidence of the magnitude of the safety consequences of the fuel rule, and a strong critique of the standard maintained by the NHTSA, see Robert W. Crandall and John D. Graham, "The Effect of Fuel Economy Standards on Automobile Safety," 32 *J. L. & Econ.* 97 (1989). See also Sam Kazman, "Death by Regulation," 14(4) *Regulation* 18 (Fall 1991).

115. For a counterexample, where an agency *did* show sensitivity to the broader effects of proposed regulations, see "FAA Decides Not to Require Safety Seat Use," *S.F. Chronicle*, Sept. 15, 1992. The Federal Aviation Administration declined to require child safety seats on airliners, reasoning that such a requirement, entailing that families would have to buy an extra ticket to accommodate the seat, would lead families to travel by road instead, where the danger of death is significantly greater. The view ultimately taken by the FAA was advocated by Sam Kazman, "Death by Regulation" (requiring child safety seats would have resulted in net loss of life). See also Richard B. McKenzie, "Making Sense of the Airline Safety Debate," 14(3) *Regulation* 76, 78 (Summer 1991) ("Air travel, measured in deaths per million miles, is more than 30 times safer than passenger-car travel").

116. See text accompanying notes 33–38.

117. Bruce N. Ames, Margie Profet, and Lois Swirsky Gold, "Dietary Pesticides (99.99% All Natural)," 87 *Proc. Nat'l Acad. Sci.* 7777 (October 1990) ("99.99 percent [by weight] of the pesticides in the American diet are chemicals that plants produce to defend themselves"). Ames has also suggested that many naturally occurring carcinogens are much more potent than the manmade chemicals currently regulated. Bruce N. Ames, Renae Magaw, and Lois Swirsky Gold, "Ranking Possible Carcinogenic Hazards," 236 *Science* 271, 276–77

(April 17, 1987). See also "Too Much Fuss about Pesticides," *Consumer Reports,* October 1989, at 655 (discussing Ames's arguments about naturally occurring pesticides).

118. See, e.g., Aaron Wildavsky, *Searching for Safety* 61–75 (1988); Aaron Wildavsky, "Richer Is Safer," 60 *The Public Interest* 23 (1980); Aaron Wildavsky, "Wealthier Is Healthier," 4(1) *Regulation,* 10 (Jan./Feb. 1980); Ralph L. Keeney, "Mortality Risks Induced by Economic Expenditures," 10 *Risk Analysis* 147, 148–49 (1990); Ralph Catalano, "The Health Effects of Economic Insecurity," 81 *Am. J. Public Health* 1148 (1991). Studies have also suggested greater cancer incidence and, more generally, lower life expectancy among those at lower socioeconomic levels. See, e.g., Claudia R. Bacquet, John W. Horm, Tyson Gibbs, and Peter Greenwald, "Socioeconomic Factors and Cancer Incidence Among Blacks and Whites," 83 *J. Nat'l Cancer Institute* 551 (1991); James S. House, Ronald C. Kessler, and A. Regula Herzog, "Age, Socioeconomic Status, and Health," 68 *Milbank Quarterly* 383 (1990).

119. Keeney, *supra* note 118, at 154–55 (citing E. M. Kitagawa and P. M. Hauser, *Differential Mortality in the United States of America: A Study in Socioeconomic Epidemiology* [1973]). The $7.25 million figure is in 1980 dollars. See also Carolyn Lochhead, "Attack on Safety Rules Begins," *S.F. Chronicle,* Mar. 24, 1992, at A2 (discussing controversy after White House endorsed consideration of such negative effects of regulatory efforts).

120. M. Harvey Brenner, "Mortality and the National Economy," *Lancet,* Sept. 15, 1979, at 568; M. Harvey Brenner, "Personal Stability and Economic Security," 8 *Social Policy* 2 (1977). See also Keeney, *supra* note 118, at 156.

121. Jack Hadley and Anthony Osei, "Does Income Affect Mortality? An Analysis of the Effects of Different Types of Income on Age/Sex/Race–Specific Mortality Rates in the United States," 20(9) *Medical Care* 901, 913 (September 1982). As a federal appeals judge noted recently, "Larger incomes can produce health by enlarging a person's access to better diet, preventive medical care, safer cars, greater leisure, etc." *International Union, U.A.W. v. O.S.H.A.,* 938 F.2d 1310, 1326 (D.C. Cir. 1991) (Williams, J., concurring separately) (citing Wildavsky, *Searching for Safety* at 59–71). See also Sylvia Nasar, "Cooling the Globe Would Be Nice, But Saving Lives Now May Cost Less," *N.Y. Times,* May 31, 1992, at D6 (discussing need for economic growth to increase income levels and so allow for financing of environmental quality controls).

122. Following the lead of the Office of Information and Regulatory Affairs (OIRA) of the Office of Management and Budget (OMB), the Occupational Safety and Health Administration (OSHA) has recently decided to study the income/health effects issue, and to "consider whether weighing the risks to workers from exposures to toxic substances with the risks associated with lowering those same workers' incomes is appropriate and relevant, and [solicit] public comment on such 'risk-risk analysis.'" Occupational Safety and Health Administration, "Air Contaminants: Proposed Rule," 57 Fed. Reg. 26002, 26006 (June

12, 1992). OSHA and OMB have also agreed that a more general look across federal agencies at the issue is merited. Letter of Nancy Risque Rohrbach, Department of Labor, to James B. McRae, Jr., OIRA, March 23, 1992; letter of James B. McRae, Jr., to Nancy Risque Rohrbach, March 24, 1992. In a thorough summary of the literature so far studied by OIRA, OSHA finds that the evidence "suggest[s] that losses in wages in the range of $1.9 million to $6.5 million dollars annually are associated with one additional fatality annually." 57 Fed. Reg. at 26006. See also Robert D. Hershey, Jr., "Citing Cost, Budget Office Blocks Workplace Health Proposal," *N.Y. Times,* March 16, 1992, at A13 (quoting James B. McRae, Jr., of the Office of Information and Regulatory Affairs: "O.S.H.A. should estimate whether the possible effect of compliance costs on workers' health will outweigh the health improvements that may result from decreased exposure to the regulated substances. In addition, the effect of higher compliance costs [and therefore lower incomes] on other members of society also should be taken into account"). In a recent concurring opinion, Judge Stephen Williams, drawing on Keeney's article cited above, explained, "Incremental safety regulation reduces incomes and thus may exact a cost in human lives. For example, if analysis showed that 'an individual life was lost for every $12 million taken from individuals [as a result of the regulation], this would be a guide to a reasonable value tradeoff for many programs designed to save lives.' Keeney, 'Mortality Risks Induced by Economic Expenditures,' 10 *Risk Analysis* at 158. Such a figure could serve as a ceiling for value-of-life calculated by other means, since regulation causing greater expenditures per life expected to be saved would, everything else being equal, result in a net *loss* of life." *International Union, U.A.W. v. O.S.H.A.,* 938 F.2d 1310, 1326–27 (D.C. Cir. 1991) (Williams, J., concurring separately). Keeney also notes that "perhaps a range of $1–25 million per life saved would be useful to appraise safety alternatives. Only in clearly justified cases would a tradeoff outside this range be used." Keeney at 158. It is interesting to compare the statistical studies showing that unions typically bargain for safety costs of $2–$10 million per life saved (note 110), with the numbers suggesting that expenditure of more than $7 million or so per statistical life saved is counterproductive (note 119). The numbers, in a sense, are consistent and can be read to suggest a rough outer bound limit of sensible expenditures. Compare the "minimum value for preventing a death" of £660,000 (about $1–1.3 million, at late-1992 rates) assigned by the English Department of Transport in 1987 and adopted by the English Health and Safety Executive in 1992. See Bronwen Maddox, "The Cost of Fear," *Financial Times,* Oct. 7, 1992, at 10; for a recent English approach to several of the issues considered in this and the next chapter, see Health and Safety Executive, *The Tolerability of Risk from Nuclear Power Stations* (HMSO, 1992).

123. See generally Michael Gough, "Estimating Risks and Ignoring Killers," paper prepared for Cato Institute conference "Making Sense of Safety," March 21–22,

1991, at 9–12 ("If we are interested in improving the health and life expectancies of poor people, we have to look at problems of society that are deeper rooted and far more intractable than reducing chemical exposures— homicides, AIDS, smoking, eating habits, and drinking. Those problems have confounded us all, but they probably offer the best opportunity to make material improvements in health and longevity").

124. Some commentators note that radon, which is estimated to lead to 10,000 to 15,000 cases of lung cancer each year, has received little notice compared to benzene or dioxin, although it causes 100 times more cancers. See, e.g., Lester B. Lave, "How Safe Is Safe Enough? Setting Safety Goals" 20 (Center for the Study of American Business, Jan. 1990). See also Christopher J. Daggett, Robert E. Hazen, and Judith Auer Shaw, "Advancing Environmental Protection through Risk Assessment," 14 *Colum. J. Envtl. L.* 315, 323 (1989) (noting how National Academy of Science's study confirmed EPA's concerns about radon, contrary to claims that the agency was overstating the risk).

125. See Michael Gough, "How Much Cancer Can EPA Regulate Away?" 10 *Risk Analysis*, 1, 6 (1990); U.S. Environmental Protection Agency, *Unfinished Business: A Comparative Assessment of Environmental Problems,* Overview Report at 62 (1987) (discussing danger of indoor pollution other than radon). See also Warren E. Leary, "New Study Offers More Evidence Linking Cancer to Halogen Lamps," *N.Y. Times,* April 16, 1992, at B6.

126. See Lester B. Lave, Fanny K. Ennever, Herbert S. Rosenkrantz, and Gilbert S. Omenn, "Information Value of the Rodent Bioassay," 336 *Nature* 631, 632 (Dec. 15, 1988) ("Devoting more resources to helping people to give up smoking or change their diet, or to screening for breast and colon cancer, would save many lives"), citing U.S. National Cancer Institute, *Cancer Goals for 2000* (Dept. of Health and Human Services, 1987); "Processors Target Diet and Cancer Connections," *Prepared Foods,* March 1991, at 40 ("an often quoted study published in 1977 . . . estimated that 40 percent of cancers among men and 60 percent of all cancers among women were diet-related").

127. Barry Commoner in *Making Peace with the Planet* (1990) urges that environmental protection must focus on prevention rather than control. See id. at 41–55.

128. Charles W. Powers, John A. Moore, and Arthur Upton, "Improving the Coherence of Federal Regulation of Risks from Hazardous Substances" 8–9 (1992) (revision of a draft paper originally prepared for the Carnegie Commission on Science, Technology and Government).

2. Causes

1. See, e.g., Leslie Roberts, "Counting on Science at the EPA," 249 *Science* 616 (Aug. 10, 1990).

2. See generally W. Lorence, *Of Acceptable Risk* (1976); Council for Science and

Society, *The Acceptability of Risks* (1977). See also National Resource Council, *Improving Risk Communication* 35 (1989); Donald T. Hornstein, "Reclaiming Environmental Law: A Normative Critique of Comparative Risk Analysis," 92 *Colum. L. Rev.* 561, 614–15 (1992); Kai Erikson, "Toxic Reckoning: Business Faces a New Kind of Fear," *Harvard Business Review* 118 (January/February 1990) (discussing society's special fear of toxic and radioactive harms); Christopher J. Daggett, Robert E. Hazen, and Judith Auer Shaw, "Advancing Environmental Protection through Risk Assessment," 14 *Colum. J. Envtl. L.* 315, 319 (1989) ("The role of the media, the effect of catastrophic events, and a general sense of lack of control all affect how the public perceives risk").

3. Baruch Fischhoff, "Risk: A Guide to Controversy," in National Resource Council, *Improving Risk Communication* 278–80 (1989).

4. See generally Baruch Fischhoff, "Managing Risk Perceptions," 2(1) *Issues in Science and Technology* 83 (National Academy of Sciences, 1985). For a discussion of how human decision making differs from the view, under conventional decision theory, that people strive to maximize expected value, see Roger G. Noll and James E. Krier, "Some Implications of Cognitive Psychology for Risk Regulation," 19 *J. Legal Stud.* 747 (1990). For suggestions that inaccurate public risk perceptions may arise rationally under conditions of uncertainty, see W. Kip Viscusi and Wesley A. Magat, *Learning about Risk: Consumer Responses to Hazard Information* 4–5 (1987) (citing W. Kip Viscusi, "A Bayesian Perspective on Biases in Risk Perception," 17 *Economics Letters* 59 [1985]); Richard A. Posner, *The Economics of Justice,* ch. 6 (1981).

5. See Baruch Fischhoff, "Managing Risk Perceptions," 2(1) *Issues in Science and Technology* 83 (National Academy of Sciences, 1985); Roger G. Noll and James E. Krier, "Some Implications of Cognitive Psychology for Risk Regulation," 19 *J. Legal Stud.* 747, 749–50, 777 (1990); Donald T. Hornstein, "Reclaiming Environmental Law: A Normative Critique of Comparative Risk Analysis," 92 *Colum. L. Rev.* 561, 605–10 (1992).

6. See generally Mary Douglas and Aaron Wildavsky, *Risk and Culture* (1982). For a classic anthropological exploration of the meanings of such ways of thinking, see Mary Douglas, *Purity and Danger: An Analysis of the Concepts of Pollution and Taboo* (1966).

7. See, e.g., Massimo Piattelli-Palmarini, "Probability Blindness: Neither Rational nor Capricious," *Bostonia* 28, 31 (March/April 1991).

8. See, e.g., Clayton P. Gillette and James E. Krier, "Risk, Courts, and Agencies," 138 *U. Penn. L. Rev.* 1027, 1033 (1990) (risk aversion of public "generally unjustified, and inconsistent with the objective of minimizing total risk costs").

9. See, e.g. Roger G. Noll and James E. Krier, "Some Implications of Cognitive Psychology for Risk Regulation," 19 *J. Legal Stud.* 747 (1990); Peter M. Sandman, "Risk Communication: Facing Public Outrage," *EPA Journal,* Nov. 1981, at 21, 22 (discussing "memorability").

10. But see an editorial by the physicist Robert L. Park, "With Alarming Frequency," *N.Y. Times,* Sept. 1, 1991, at E11 ("Some of the coverage [of health risks] will be excessively sensational, but the media will not and should not wait for scientists to give the all-clear. What should be given greater emphasis is the scientist's obligation to try to put the risk in proper perspective for the public").

11. See Gideon Koren and Naomi Klein, "Bias against Negative Studies in Newspaper Reports of Medical Research," 266 *JAMA* 1824 (October 2, 1991); see also Richard Knox, "Study Finds Vitamin D Helps Slow Bone Loss," *Boston Globe,* Oct. 3, 1991, at 3 (discussing *JAMA* study).

12. For a broad discussion of the disputes between experts and the public, see Baruch Fischhoff, "Risk: A Guide to Controversy," in National Resource Council, *Improving Risk Communication* 272–281 (1989). See also National Resource Council, *Improving Risk Communication* 70 (1989) (noting public's distrust of experts).

13. Baruch Fischhoff, "Managing Risk Perceptions," 2(1) *Issues in Science and Technology* 83, 88 (1985). See also Cristine Russell, "What, Me Worry?" *American Health* 45, 49 (June 1990); see generally Roger G. Noll and James E. Krier, "Some Implications of Cognitive Psychology for Risk Regulation," 19 *J. Legal Stud.* 747, 758, 771 (1990).

14. Kevin McKean, "Decisions, Decisions," in *Discover,* June 1985, at 22; Massimo Piattelli-Palmarini, "Probability Blindness: Neither Rational nor Capricious," *Bostonia* 28, 30–31 (March/April 1991) (providing similar examples); see also Baruch Fischhoff, "Risk: A Guide to Controversy," in National Resource Council, *Improving Risk Communication* 226–33 (1989); Amos Tversky and Daniel Kahneman, "Rational Choice and the Framing of Decisions," 59 *J. Business* S251 (1986). Cf. John Tierney, "Behind Monty Hall's Doors: Puzzle, Debate and Answer?" *N.Y. Times,* July 21, 1991, §1, at 1 (even experts get it wrong when picking doors on "Let's Make a Deal"); Roger G. Noll and James E. Krier, "Some Implications of Cognitive Psychology for Risk Regulation," 19 *J. Legal Stud.* 747, 768 (1990) (voters' evaluation of policy options will be affected by the way political actors describe issues).

15. See McKean, "Decisions, Decisions," at 25; see also Baruch Fischhoff, "Risk: A Guide to Controversy," in National Resource Council, *Improving Risk Communication* 248 (1989).

16. Letter from Oliver Wendell Holmes, Jr. to Canon Patrick Augustine Sheehan (July 5, 1912), in *Holmes-Sheehan Letters: The Letters of Justice Oliver Wendell Holmes and Canon Patrick Augustine Sheehan* 45 (David H. Burton, ed. 1976). "Experts" themselves are, of course, not immune from such pitfalls. See *infra,* note 56. Moreover, there is some debate over whether such ways of thinking on the part of the general public are really irrational or, rather, should be accorded more respect by experts in risk assessment. See Paul Slovic, "Percep-

tion of Risk," 236 *Science* 280, 284–85 (April 17, 1987) ("Lay people some-times lack certain information about hazards. However, their basic conceptuali-zation of risk is much richer than that of the experts and reflects legitimate concerns that are typically omitted from expert risk assessments. . . . Each side, expert and public, has something valid to contribute"); Donald T. Hornstein, "Reclaiming Environmental Law: A Normative Critique of Comparative Risk Analysis," 92 *Colum. L. Rev.* 561, 610–11 and n.228 (1992); Peter M. Sandman, "Risk Communication: Facing Public Outrage," *EPA Journal,* Nov. 1981, at 21, 22 ("we have *two decades of data* indicating that voluntariness, control, fairness, and the rest are important components of our society's definition of risk. When a risk manager continues to ignore these factors—and continues to be surprised by the public's response of outrage—it is worth asking just whose behavior is irrational") (emphasis in original).

17. See Robert A. Hamilton, "Country Club Workers Are Lucky Twice," *N.Y. Times,* Jan. 25, 1987, §11CN, at 3.

18. For discussion of these effects in reference to Love Canal, see Aaron Wildavsky, "If Claims of Harm from Technology Are False, Mostly False, or Unproven, What Does That Tell Us about Science?" in *Health, Lifestyle, and Environment: Countering the Panic* 111, 112–14 (Social Affairs Unit, Manhattan Institute, 1991). Note that the unequally dramatic quality of various risks leads not only to overregulation, but also to underregulation of more "mundane" risks: see Adam M. Finkel, "Is Risk Assessment Really Too Conservative? Revising the Revisionists," 14 *Colum. J. Envtl. L.* 427, 458 (1989).

19. See, e.g., Bernard L. Cohen and I-Sing Lee, "A Catalog of Risks," 36 *Health Physics* 707, 718 (1979) (noting how catastrophic events frequently receive a great deal of publicity, even where no deaths are involved).

20. See National Resource Council, *Improving Risk Communication* 18 (1989); William D. Ruckelshaus, "Risk, Science, and Democracy," 2(1) *Issues in Science and Technology,* 33–34 (National Academy of Sciences, 1985).

21. Baruch Fischhoff, "Managing Risk Perceptions," 2(1) *Issues in Science and Technology* 83, 86 (National Academy of Sciences, 1985).

22. See generally Matthew L. Wald, "As Science Gauges Perils in Life, To Learn More Is to Know Less," *N.Y. Times,* Aug. 19, 1991, at A1; Cyril L. Comar, "Introduction, Risk: A Pragmatic De Minimis Approach," in *De Minimis Risk* xiii (Chris Whipple, ed., 1987).

23. See J. N. Kapferer, "A Mass Poisoning Rumor in Europe," 53 *Public Opinion Quarterly* 467 (1989).

24. See generally Wildavsky, "If Claims of Harm from Technology Are False"; Peter W. Huber, *Galileo's Revenge: Junk Science in the Courtroom,* chs. 4, 10 (1991). See also Andrea Arnold, *Fear of Food: Environmentalist Scams, Media Men-dacity, and the Law of Disparagement* (1990); "Educational Group Warns against Emphasis on Environmental Pollution as Cancer Cause," in 16 *Environ-ment Reporter* 1093 (BNA, October 25, 1985); Robert James Bidinotto, "The

Great Apple Scare," in *Reader's Digest* 53 (October 1990) (discussing Alar panic). But see Adrian De Wind, "Alar's Gone, Little Thanks to the Government," *N.Y. Times,* July 30, 1991, at A18 (letter to editor, disputing claims that Alar was not particularly harmful, and that its ban harmed the apple industry without real benefit to the public).

25. 42 U.S.C. §9621(d)(1), (2)(A); emphasis added.

26. See Environmental Protection Agency, "National Oil and Hazardous Substances Pollution Contingency Plan," 55 Fed. Reg. 8666 (1990); Lawrence E. Starfield, "The 1990 National Contingency Plan—More Detail and More Structure, but Still a Balancing Act," 20 *Envtl. L. Rep.* 10222 (1990).

27. See Dave Willis, "Rational Regulation of Risk," (student seminar paper at the John F. Kennedy School of Government) 3–5 (1991) (citations omitted).

28. See R. Shep Melnick, "The Politics of Benefit-Cost Analysis," in P. Brett Hammond and Rob Coppock, eds., *Valuing Health Risks, Costs, and Benefits for Environmental Decision Making: Report of a Conference* (1990) at 23.

29. Indeed, John Mendeloff has found that "of the dozens of oversight hearings on health and safety, 'all but four featured criticisms that agencies had been too lax.'" Quoted in Melnick, id. at 32.

30. 21 U.S.C. §348(c)(3)(A); *Les v. Reilly,* 968 F.2d 985, 986 (9th Cir.), petition for cert. filed (Nov. 6, 1992) (interpreting Delaney clause as prohibiting use of four pesticides which EPA found to be carcinogens as food additives even where cancer risk they posed was "de minimis"; Delaney clause "prohibit[s] all additives that are carcinogens, regardless of the degree of risk involved").

31. 42 U.S.C. §6924(d)(1). See also Erik H. Corwin, "Congressional Limits on Agency Discretion: A Case Study of the Hazardous and Solid Waste Amendments of 1984," 29 *Harv. J. on Legis.* 517, 534–35 (1992); William L. Rosbe and Robert L. Gulley, "The Hazardous and Solid Waste Amendments of 1984: A Dramatic Overhaul of the Way America Manages Its Hazardous Wastes," 14 *Envtl. L. Rep.* 10458 (1984).

32. 42 U.S.C. §6924(d),(e). See generally Walter E. Mugdan and Bruce R. Adler, "The 1984 RCRA Amendments: Congress as a Regulatory Agency," 10 *Colum. J. Envtl. L.* 215 (1985).

33. See 42 U.S.C. §6924(g)(6).

34. See 42 U.S.C. §7412(f)(2)(A).

35. See Erik H. Corwin, "Congressional Limits on Agency Discretion: A Case Study of the Hazardous and Solid Waste Amendments of 1984," 29 *Harv. J. on Legis.* 517, 542–49 (1992).

36. Id. at 531–33; Sam Kazman, "Death by Regulation," 14(4) *Regulation* 18, 18 (Fall 1991).

37. See R. Shep Melnick, "The Politics of Benefit-Cost Analysis," in P. Brett Hammond and Rob Coppock, eds., *Valuing Health Risks, Costs, and Benefits for Environmental Decision Making: Report of a Conference* (1990) at 23.

38. See John V. Tunney, "The Federal Legislative Process: Misinformation, Reac-

tion, and Excessive Delegation," 7 *Envtl. L.* 499 (1977) (arguing that major regulatory efforts between 1962 and 1976 responded to perceived crises, that these efforts paid little attention to cost-benefit analyses of issues, and that Congressmen generally did not know what they were voting on).

39. Cf. Baruch Fischhoff, "Risk: A Guide to Controversy," in National Resource Council, *Improving Risk Communication* 240–42 (1989).

40. Id. at 244–45 (noting how "even sophisticated individuals have poor intuitions about the size of the sample needed to test research hypotheses accurately"); id. at 217 ("science of risk" "depends on the educated intuitions of scientists, rather than on accepted hard facts; although these may be the judgments of trained experts, they still need to be recognized as matters of conjecture that are both more likely to be overturned than published [and replicated] results and more vulnerable to the vagaries of the psychological process").

41. For a discussion of overspending on the illusion of greater safety in an engineering context, see Lester B. Lave, Daniel Resendiz-Carrillo, and Francis C. McMichael, "Safety Goals for High-Hazard Dams: Are Dams Too Safe?" 26 *Water Resources Research* 1383 (July 1990).

42. See Lester B. Lave, "How Safe Is Safe Enough? Setting Safety Goals" 7 (Center for the Study of American Business, Jan. 1990).

43. See Stephen Breyer, *Regulation and Its Reform* 136–37 (1982) (discussing difficulties with prospective studies).

44. See id. at 137 (discussing difficulties with retrospective studies); W. Kip Viscusi, *Risk by Choice: Regulating Health Safety in the Workplace* 60–63 (1983).

45. Animal studies are also often criticized as expensive and uninformative. See, e.g., Lester B. Lave, Fanny K. Ennever, Herbert S. Rosenkrantz, and Gilbert S. Omenn, "Information Value of the Rodent Bioassay," 336 *Nature* 631 (Dec. 15, 1988) ("We find that the bioassay often does not provide information commensurate with its cost, implying that the regulatory policies of industrialized countries need to be changed").

46. In 1985, the federal Office of Science and Technology Policy wrote, "models . . . which incorporate low-dose linearity are preferred when compatible with the limited information." Principle 26, Office of Science and Technology Policy Cancer Principles (U.S. Interagency Staff Group on Carcinogens, Feb. 1985), reprinted in Federal Focus, Inc., *Toward Common Measures: Recommendations for a Presidential Executive Order in Environmental Risk Assessment and Risk Management Policy* 129 (1991). But see *infra* note 48.

47. See Matthew L. Wald, "As Science Gauges Perils in Life, to Learn More Is to Know Less," *N.Y. Times,* Aug. 19, 1991, at A1, A11 (providing similar hypothetical).

48. The American Council on Science and Health noted in 1990 that an assumption of linearity (that there is no threshold below which the substance is not harmful) is not scientifically "tenable." American Council on Science and Health, "From Mice to Men," in *The Benefits and Limitations of Animal Testing in Predicting*

Human Cancer Risk 21–33 (1990). See also the letter from Frederica P. Perera and the response of Bruce Ames and Lois Gold, "Carcinogens and Human Health: Part 1," 250 *Science* 1644 (Dec. 21, 1990) (disputing validity of low-dose linearity assumption); Albert N. Nichols and Richard J. Zeckhauser, "The Perils of Prudence: How Conservative Risk Assessments Distort Regulation," *Regulation* 13, 16 (November/December 1986) (noting "heroic" assumptions in dose-response analyses); Federal Focus, Inc., *Toward Common Measures: Recommendations for a Presidential Executive Order in Environmental Risk Assessment and Risk Management Policy* 75–78 (1991). But cf. Matthew L. Wald, "As Science Gauges Perils in Life, to Learn More Is to Know Less," *N.Y. Times,* Aug. 19, 1991, at A1, A11 (quoting David Doniger of Natural Resources Defense Council: "If you don't really know, if you have a wide range, the only prudent thing to do in public health is to be safe rather than sorry"—that is, to use the linear, no-threshold model).

49. See John D. Graham, "Improving Chemical Risk Assessment," 14(4) *Regulation* 14, 16–17 (Fall 1991).

50. See *Health Effects of Exposure to Low Levels of Ionizing Radiation, Bier V* 26–29 (National Research Council 1990); Arthur C. Upton, "Carcinogenic Effects of Low-Level Ionizing Radiation," 82 *J. National Cancer Institute* 448 (March 21, 1990); *The Effects on Populations of Exposure to Low Levels of Ionizing Radiation: 1980* 142–47 (National Research Council 1980); see also Ching-Hon Pui et al., "Acute Myeloid Leukemia in Children Treated with Epipodophyllotoxins for Acute Lymphoblastic Leukemia," 325 *New Eng. J. Medicine* 1682 (Dec. 12, 1991) (discussing relationship between dose and schedule of epipodophyllotoxins and development of secondary acute myeloid leukemia).

51. For a critique, see Bruce N. Ames, Renae Magaw, and Lois Swirsky Gold, "Ranking Possible Carcinogenic Hazards," in 236 *Science* 271, 275–276 (April 17, 1987). But see Werner K. Lutz, "Dose-Response Relationship and Low Dose Extrapolation in Chemical Carcinogenesis," 11 *Carcinogenesis* 1243 (1990) (suggesting that for heterogenous human populations, linear or near-linear curves may often be appropriate); Frederica P. Perera, "Carcinogens and Human Health: Part 1," 250 *Science* 1644 (Dec. 21, 1990) (letter to the editor criticizing Ames et al., and suggesting that linear dose/response assumptions are often appropriate). Cf. Bruce N. Ames and Lois S. Gold, "Carcinogens and Human Health: Part 1," 250 *Science* 1645 (Dec. 21, 1990) (letter to the editor, responding to Perera).

52. See, e.g., Department of Labor, "Occupational Exposure to Benzene," 52 Fed. Reg. 34460, 34490–91 (linear dose/response curve determined regulatory outcome).

53. See Wildavsky, "If Claims of Harm from Technology Are False," 111, 124 n.28, quoting D. A. Freedman and H. Zeisel, "From Mouse-to-Man: The Quantitative Assessment of Cancer Risks," 3 *Statistical Science* 3, 6 (1988).

54. See Albert N. Nichols and Richard J. Zeckhauser, "The Perils of Prudence: How Conservative Risk Assessments Distort Regulation," *Regulation* 13, 16 (November/December 1986).

55. Cf. Glenna M. Kyle, "A Legal and Scientific Critique of the Use of Animal Data in Proving Causation," in 1 *Courts, Health Science, and the Law* 429 (1991) (arguing for courts to exercise caution in admitting extrapolation data in court).

56. Moreover, evidence suggests that experts have their own biases in the risk assessment process: they may test and retest until they get positive results; they may not fully understand the low predictive power of small samples; they may become overconfident. See, e.g., Baruch Fischhoff, "Risk: A Guide to Controversy," in National Resource Council, *Improving Risk Communication* 244–45 (1989). Experts may also often be prey to the same cognitive tendencies that dog the lay public. Amos Tversky, a leading cognitive psychologist who studies decision theory, has noted, "Whenever you find an error that statistically naive people make, you can find a more sophisticated version of the same problem that will trip the experts." Kevin McKean, "Decisions, Decisions," *Discover,* June 1985, at 22, 31. See also Paul Slovic, "Perception of Risk," 236 *Science* 280, 281 (April 17, 1987) ("experts' judgments appear to be prone to many of the same biases as those of the general public") (citing sources).

57. See Albert L. Nichols and Richard J. Zeckhauser, "The Perils of Prudence: How Conservative Risk Assessments Distort Regulation," in *Regulation* 13 (Nov./Dec. 1986); see also Adam M. Finkel, *Confronting Uncertainty in Risk Management: A Guide for Decision-Makers* (Resources for the Future, 1990); George M. Gray and John D. Graham, "Risk Assessment and Clean Air Policy," 10 *Journal of Policy Analysis and Management* 286 (1991). See also Dale Hattis and Robert L. Goble, "Expected Values for Projected Cancer Risks from Putative Genetically Acting Agents," 11 *Risk Analysis* 359 (1991) (discussing "upper confidence limits" and alternative models for communicating risk levels).

58. See Lester B. Lave, Fanny K. Ennever, Herbert S. Rosenkrantz, and Gilbert S. Omenn, "Information Value of the Rodent Bioassay," 336 *Nature* 631, 631 (Dec. 15, 1988) ("Rats and mice are more similar biologically to each other than either is to humans"). Holmes Rolston has likened formal risk analysis to weighing hogs in Texas: "Down there, they put the hog in one pan of a large set of scales, put rocks in the other pan, one by one, until they exactly balance the weight of the hog. Having done that very carefully, they guess how much the rocks weigh." Quoted in K. S. Shrader-Frechette, *Science, Policy, Ethics, and Economic Methodology* 48 (1985).

59. See generally Bruce N. Ames, Renae Magaw, and Lois Swirsky Gold, "Ranking Possible Carcinogenic Hazards," 236 *Science* 271, 275–76 (April 17, 1987) (summarizing uncertainties); Albert N. Nichols and Richard J. Zeckhauser, "The Perils of Prudence: How Conservative Risk Assessments Distort Regulation," *Regulation* 13, 17 (November/December 1986). But cf. David P. Rall, "Carcinogens and Human Health: Part 2," 251 *Science* 10 (Jan. 4, 1991)

(suggesting that animal studies remain a useful tool for identifying potentially hazardous compounds).

60. Bruce N. Ames, Renae Magaw, and Lois Swirsky Gold, "Ranking Possible Carcinogenic Hazards," 236 *Science* 271, 276 (April 17, 1987); Jean Marx, "Animal Carcinogen Testing Challenged," 250 *Science* 743 (Nov. 9, 1990) (discussing controversy over Ames's criticism of animal studies). See also Richard B. Belzer, "The Peril and Promise of Risk Assessment," 14(4) *Regulation* 40, 42–43 (Fall 1991); OMB, *Regulatory Program of the United States Government, April 1, 1990–March 31, 1991,* at 18 ("It is therefore unclear whether the cancers induced are caused by formaldehyde per se or by the toxic effects of high doses"). But cf. I. Bernard Weinstein, "Mitogenesis Is Only One Factor in Carcinogenesis," 251 *Science* 387 (Jan. 25, 1991) (disputing claims of Ames et al., and suggesting that rodent bioassays remain very helpful).

61. See, e.g., Bruce C. Allen, Kenny S. Crump, and Annette M. Shipp, "Correlation between Carcinogenic Potency of Chemicals in Animals and Humans," 8 *Risk Analysis* 531 (1988); John C. Bailar III, Edmund A. C. Crouch, Rashid Shaikh, and Donna Spiegelman, "One-Hit Models of Carcinogenesis: Conservative or Not?" 8 *Risk Analysis* 485 (1988).

62. Bruce N. Ames, Renae Magaw, and Lois Swirsky Gold, "Ranking Possible Carcinogenic Hazards," 236 *Science* 271, 274 (April 17, 1987); *Regulatory Program of the United States Government, April 1, 1990–March 31, 1991,* at 19 ("formaldehyde causes nasal tumors in rats at 12 times the rate observed in the next most sensitive animal species. This extreme sensitivity may be related to the fact that rats breathe only through the nose"). "Rats, unlike humans, are obligate nose breathers." John D. Graham, Laura C. Green, and Marc J. Roberts, *In Search of Safety: Chemicals and Cancer Risk* 183 (1988).

63. See, e.g., Bruce N. Ames, Renae Magaw, and Lois Swirsky Gold, "Ranking Carcinogenic Hazards," 17 *Science* 271, 275 (1985) (humans live longer).

64. "For example, some chemicals cause cancer in the zymbal gland of the rat; because humans lack such a gland it is unclear whether these results matter in estimating human health risk." *Regulatory Program of the United States Government, April 1, 1990–March 31, 1991,* at 19.

65. See, e.g., John D. Graham, "Improving Chemical Risk Assessment," 14(4) *Regulation* 14, 17 (Fall 1991); Charles W. Powers, John A. Moore, and Arthur Upton, "Improving the Coherence of Federal Regulation of Risks from Hazardous Substances" 22 n.22 (1992) (revision of a draft paper originally prepared for the Carnegie Commission on Science, Technology and Government). For a discussion of transport of toxic chemicals in the various human systems, see generally Morton Lippmann, "Toxic Chemical Exposure and Dose to Target Tissues," in *Toxic Chemicals, Health, and the Environment* 114 (Lester B. Lave and Arthur C. Upton, eds., 1987).

66. See, e.g., Bruce N. Ames, Renae Magaw, and Lois Swirsky Gold, "Ranking Possible Carcinogenic Hazards," 236 *Science* 271, 273, Table 1 (April 17, 1987).

67. See Graham, "Improving Chemical Risk Assessment."
68. Richard B. Belzer, "The Peril and Promise of Risk Assessment," 14(4) *Regulation* 40, 45 (Fall 1991) ("Occupational cancer risks are based on . . . a hypothetical worker who is exposed at the permissible exposure limit eight hours per day, five days per week, fifty weeks per year over a forty-five-year working lifetime").
69. Id. at 40, 46. For critiques of such exposure assumptions in the EPA, see Robert H. Harris and David E. Burmaster, "Restoring Science to Superfund Risk Assessment," 6 *Toxics Law Reporter* 1318 (1992) (analyzing EPA procedures which purport to yield estimates of the 90th to 95th percentile exposure and concluding that those procedures yield estimates in excess of the 99th percentile exposure, exceeding the best 95th percentile exposure estimate by factors of up to 500); Graham, "Improving Chemical Risk Assessment," 14, 15: "EPA now needs to . . . replace unrealistic exposure assessments with available data about factors such as population mobility, facility lifetime, indoor versus outdoor sources of pollutants, and the amount of time spent indoors and outdoors." See also Albert N. Nichols and Richard J. Zeckhauser, "The Perils of Prudence: How Conservative Risk Assessments Distort Regulation," *Regulation* 13, 15 (November/December 1986).
70. "Suppose that there are ten independent steps in a risk assessment and prudence dictates assumptions that in each instance result in risk estimates two times the expected value. Such a process would yield a summary risk estimate that is more than 1,000 times higher than the most likely risk estimate. Because there are usually many more than ten steps, and many of them will incorporate conservative biases that exceed [that] order of magnitude, risk estimates based on such practices will often exceed the most likely value by a factor of one million or more." OMB, *Regulatory Program of the United States, April 1, 1990–March 31, 1991* 26. See also id. at 22, 23 (EPA, CDC, and FDA risk assessments for dioxins exceed those adopted by other governments by a factor of a thousand, and exceed the "most likely estimate" by a factor of 5,000; "plausible estimates for perchloroethylene . . . vary by a factor of about 35,000").
71. More recent risk analysis often takes account of the effects of multiple pathways. See Richard B. Belzer, "The Peril and Promise of Risk Assessment," 14(4) *Regulation* 40, 46 (Fall 1991).
72. See generally Albert N. Nichols and Richard J. Zeckhauser, "The Perils of Prudence: How Conservative Risk Assessments Distort Regulation," *Regulation* 13 (November/December 1986).
73. See generally Adam M. Finkel, "Is Risk Assessment Really Too Conservative? Revising the Revisionists," 14 *Colum. J. Envtl. L.* 427, 432–34, 443–47, 449–53 (1989). Finkel also notes that such apparently conservative assumptions as linear dose extrapolation models can sometimes yield serious underestimates of risks. Id. at 443.
74. Cf. id. at 461.

75. See, e.g., Philip H. Abelson, "Exaggerated Carcinogenicity of Chemicals," 256 *Science* 1609 (June 19, 1992) (noting cumulative biases in risk assessment models for butadiene); Albert N. Nichols and Richard J. Zeckhauser, "The Perils of Prudence: How Conservative Risk Assessments Distort Regulation," *Regulation* 13 (November/December 1986) ("The cumulative effect of . . . using a long series of conservative assumptions, can be monumental overestimates of health risks. The result is a more stringent and costly regulation of at least some types of risk than if policy makers were fully informed"). But see Adam M. Finkel, "Is Risk Assessment Really Too Conservative? Revising the Revisionists," 14 *Colum. J. Envtl. L.* 427, 447–48 (1989) (urging caution, in the light of pervasive uncertainties, against the assumption that multiple apparently conservative steps will necessarily lead to gross exaggerations of risk).

76. See generally Richard Wilson and E. A. C. Crouch, "Risk Assessment and Comparisons: An Introduction," 236 *Science* 267, 270 (April 17, 1987) ("It is important to realize that risks appear to be very different when expressed in different ways. . . . Of course, none of the methods of expressing the risk can be considered 'right' in an absolute sense") (citations omitted); see also George M. Gray and John D. Graham, "Risk Assessment and Clean Air Policy," 10 *J. Policy Analysis & Mgmt.* 286 (1991) (discussing how executive summaries of risk assessments may distort actual findings).

77. See "Immediate Suspension of EDB for Fumigation of Grain Issued; Other Restrictions Initiated," in 14 *Environment Reporter* 1757 (BNA, February 10, 1984).

78. See, e.g., "California Adopts Plan to Ban EDB in Shelf-Food Products by July 1, 1985," in 14 *Environment Reporter* 2197 (BNA, March 30, 1984).

79. Harold Issadore Sharlin, "Macro-Risks, Micro-Risks, and the Media: The EDB Case," in *The Social and Cultural Construction of Risk* 183, 186 (B. B. Johnson and V. T. Covello, eds. 1987).

80. Id. at 192, quoting the Dallas *Morning News,* Jan. 8, 1984 (quoting EPA Administrator William D. Ruckelshaus).

81. Id. at 192–93.

82. Leslie Roberts, "Counting on Science at EPA," 249 *Science* 616 (1990) ("The agencies' budgets and priorities have been shaped more by 'what the last phone call from Capitol Hill or the last public opinion poll had to say' than by scientific assessment of risk, says [an official] of EPA's office of policy analysis"). For a description of a particulary politicized period at the EPA, see Joel M. Mintz, "Agencies, Congress, and Regulatory Enforcement: A Review of the EPA's Hazardous Waste Enforcement Effort, 1970–1987," 18 *Envtl. L.* 683, 715–743, 751–759 (1988) (describing the disarray and Congressional response during the "Burford" years, 1981–1983).

83. Commentators have also noted how political considerations may influence the assumptions and procedures of scientists and technical specialists, affecting the outcome of supposedly scientific analyses. See, e.g., John C. Bailar III and

Stephen R. Thomas, "What Are We Doing When We Think We Are Doing Risk Analysis?" in *Assessment of Risk from Low-level Exposure to Radiation and Chemicals: A Critical Overview,* 65, 68 (Avril D. Woodhead et al. eds., 1985) (vol. 33 of the Basic Life Sciences series).

84. The effects of OMB review are discussed in Chapter 3.

85. See Jerry L. Mashaw and David L. Harfst, *The Struggle for Auto Safety,* ch. 8 (1990); Thomas O. McGarity, "Thoughts on 'Deossifying' the Rulemaking Process," 1–18, 32–34, discussion draft prepared for the meeting of the Carnegie Commission Task Force on Science and Technology in Judicial and Regulatory Decision Making, May 24, 1991; Stephen Breyer and Richard Stewart, *Administrative Law and Regulatory Policy* 606–609 (3d ed. 1992).

86. According to John Mendeloff, one of the techniques used by agencies to avoid overregulation is "refusing to admit that a substance is potentially dangerous because the regulatory consequences of making this admission are so draconian." R. Shep Melnick, "The Politics of Benefit-Cost Analysis," in P. Brett Hammond and Rob Coppock, *Valuing Health Risks, Costs, and Benefits for Environmental Decision Making: Report of a Conference* (1990) at 23, 50, citing J. Mendeloff, "Regulatory Reform and OSHA Policy," 5 *J. Policy Analysis & Mgmt.* 440 (1986); J. Mendeloff, *The Dilemma of Toxic Substance Regulation: How Overregulation Causes Underregulation at OSHA* (1988).

87. See generally Thomas O. McGarity, "Thoughts on 'Deossifying' the Rulemaking Process," discussion draft prepared for the meeting of the Carnegie Commission Task Force on Science and Technology in Judicial and Regulatory Decision Making, May 24, 1991; Stephen Breyer and Richard Stewart, *Administrative Law and Regulatory Policy* (3d ed. 1992).

88. Previous commentators have observed the tendency of public apprehension, Congressional action, and regulatory practices to reinforce each other. For a concise discussion, see Lester B. Lave and Eric H. Malès, "At Risk: The Framework for Regulating Toxic Substances," 23 *Envtl. Sci. & Tech.* 386, 386–87 (1989).

3. Solutions

1. "Fundamental changes in concepts, in laws, and in the organizational structure of legislative and executive branch activities are essential if further progress is to be made on long-standing environmental issues and newly recognized ones alike." William K. Reilly, Jr., "A View toward the Nineties," in P. Borelli, *Crossroads: Environmental Priorities for the Future* 97 (1988), quoted in Carnegie Commission on Science, Technology, and Government, E^3: *Organizing for Environment, Energy, and the Economy in the Executive Branch of the U.S. Government* 5 (April 1990).

2. Compare Stephen Breyer, *Regulation and Its Reform,* chs. 11, 16 (1982).

3. See Chapter 2, text accompanying notes 1–38; see also Jerome J. Ravetz,

"Public Perceptions of Acceptable Risks as Evidence for Their Cognitive, Technological, and Social Structure," in *Technological Risk* 45, 46–52 (Meinoff Dierkes, Sam Edwards, and Rob Coppock, eds., 1980) (describing difficulties of achieving public consensus on acceptance of risks, in light of immaturity of relevant sciences and resulting lack of legitimacy of expert statements that certain risks are minimal or acceptable); but cf. Richard J. Zeckhauser and W. Kip Viscusi, "Risk within Reason," 248 *Science* 559, 563 (May 4, 1990) (suggesting that individuals must take increased responsibility for risk-related choices such as diet and driving habits).

4. See, e.g., *Regulatory Program of the United States Government, April 1, 1990– March 31, 1991*, at 30–32.

5. See, e.g., Paul R. Portney, "EPA and the Evolution of Federal Regulation," in *EPA and the Evolution of Federal Regulation* 17–19 (Paul R. Portney, ed., Resources for the Future, 1990) (generally discussing pros and cons of pollution tax and pollution permits).

6. Breyer, *Regulation and Its Reform,* at 161–71 (describing disclosure and taxes as alternatives to classical regulation).

7. Thomas O. McGarity, "Risk and Trust: The Role of Regulatory Agencies," in 16 *Envtl. L. Rep.* 10198, 10199 (August 1986).

8. See, e.g., R. Shep Melnick, "The Politics of Benefit-Cost Analysis," in P. Brett Hammond and Rob Coppock, *Valuing Health Risks, Costs, and Benefits for Environmental Decision Making: Report of a Conference* at 23. Compare, e.g., Michael J. Malbin, "Congress, Policy Analysis, and Natural Gas Deregulation: A Parable about Fig Leaves," in *Bureaucrats, Policy Analysts, Statesmen: Who Leads?* 62 (Robert A. Goldwin, ed., 1980) (describing limited impact, misunderstanding, and misuse to "play to the press galleries" of divergent scientific studies of natural gas deregulation); Carnegie Commission on Science, Technology, and Government, Science Technology, and Congress: *Analysis and Advice from the Congressional Support Agencies* (1991) (arguing for improvements in and expanded resources for science and technology-related support staffs for Congress as vital to "quality of congressional decisions").

9. See, e.g., *Continental Airlines, Inc. v. U.S. Dep't of Transp.,* 856 F.2d 209, 215–16 (D.C. Cir. 1988) (enforcing statutory requirement that Department of Transportation issue final order within 90 days after ALJ decision or issue ALJ decision as its own, and rejecting DOT's attempt to "escape this obligation by post hoc recharacterization of the nature of the proceedings"); *Natural Resources Defense Council v. Thomas,* 805 F.2d 410, 435 (D.C. Cir. 1986) (court has "no alternative but to enforce" Congress's "explicit leadtime requirement" for EPA promulgation of automobile emissions standards); *In re Center for Auto Safety,* 793 F.2d 1346, 1353–54 (D.C. Cir. 1986) (noting Congress's "specific deadline" for NHTSA to promulgate fuel economy standards for light trucks and NHTSA's repeated failure to meet the deadline, and "retain[ing] jurisdiction

over this case until agency publication" of current standards to "ensure future compliance with the statute").

10. 5 U.S.C. §706(2)(A).

11. See Chapter 1, text accompanying notes 42–49. For another example of a court catching an "outlier" case, where an agency decision makes no sense, see *Aqua Slide 'n' Dive Corp. v. C.P.S.C.,* 569 F.2d 831 (5th Cir. 1978) (holding that no substantial evidence supported CPSC's safety standard for swimming pool slides). Agency-specific statutes sometimes provide for a somewhat "harder look" at agency actions. *See AFL-CIO v. OSHA,* 965 F.2d 962 (11th Cir. 1992) (overturning OSHA standards for workplace exposure to pollutants because OSHA failed to offer "substantial evidence," a standard of review less deferential than APA "arbitrary and capricious review" and required by 29 U.S.C. §665(f), that the old standards permitted harmful levels or that the new standards eliminated or reduced the risk to the extent feasible, as OSHA's statute requires). See also Devra Lee Davis, "The 'Shotgun Wedding' of Science and Law: Risk Assessment and Judicial Review," 10 *Colum. J. Envtl. L.* 67, 98 (1985) (concluding that the standard of review formally applied does not determine courts' degree of scrutiny of agency's risk assessment).

12. See Stephen Breyer and Richard Stewart, *Administrative Law and Regulatory Policy,* ch. 4 (3d ed. 1992).

13. Cf. *Heckler v. Chaney,* 470 U.S. 821, 831–32 (1985) ("The agency is far better equipped than the courts to deal with the many variables involved in the proper ordering of its priorities").

14. Indeed, in reviewing administrative decisions, the courts generally are limited to the record developed before the agency. See, e.g., *Camp v. Pitts,* 411 U.S. 138, 142 (1973); *Valley Citizens for a Safe Environment v. Aldridge,* 886 F.2d 458, 459–60 (1st Cir. 1989) (explaining reasons for courts' reliance on administrative record, and describing circumstances warranting consideration of additional evidence).

15. Stephen Breyer, "The Donahue Lecture Series: 'Administering Justice in the First Circuit,'" 24 *Suffolk U. L. Rev.* 29, 33 (1990).

16. See Stephen Breyer, "Judicial Review of Questions of Law and Policy," 38 *Admin. L. Rev.* 363, 389 (1986). On the weaknesses of courts in assessing risk, see Clayton P. Gillette and James E. Krier, "Risk, Courts, and Agencies," 138 *U. Penn. L. Rev.* 1027, 1042–58 (1990).

17. *Gulf South Insulation v. United States Consumer Product Safety Commission,* 701 F.2d 1137 (5th Cir. 1983).

18. See generally Terrence M. Scanlon and Robert A. Rogowsky, "Back-Door Rulemaking: A View from the CPSC," 8(4) *Regulation* 27 (July/Aug. 1984) (describing the CPSC's preference for informally negotiated product recalls over rulemaking as prescribed in various CPSC statutes); Antonin Scalia, "Back to Basics: Making Law without Making Rules," 5(4) *Regulation* 25 (July/Aug. 1981).

19. *Corrosion Proof Fittings v. E.P.A.,* 947 F.2d 1201, 1217 (5th Cir. 1991).

20. See, e.g., Stephen Breyer and Richard Stewart, *Administrative Law and Regulatory Policy* 378–81 (3d ed., 1992), discussing *Motor Vehicle Manufacturers Ass'n v. State Farm Mutual Automobile Ins. Co.,* 463 U.S. 29, 46–56 (1983) (where it was held arbitrary and capricious for NHTSA not to have considered airbags or to have adequately considered automatic safety belts in deciding to rescind passive restraint standard). For an example of an unproductive dispute about alternatives, see *International Brotherhood of Teamsters v. U.S.,* 735 F.2d 1525 (D.C. Cir. 1984), discussed in Stephen Breyer, "Judicial Review of Questions of Law and Policy," 38 *Ad. L. Rev.* 363, 391–93 (1986). But contrast *Competitive Enterprise Inst. v. NHTSA,* 956 F.2d 321 (D.C. Cir. 1992), where the remand to the agency for "reasoned decisionmaking" (id. at 327) seems a useful way to force the agency to face crucial and inescapable choices about safety.

21. Letter from Richard A. Merrill to the author, March 23, 1992. See also Jerry Mashaw and David Harfst, "Regulation and Legal Culture: The Case of Motor Vehicle Safety," 4 *Yale J. on Reg.* 258, 295 (1987) ("Any remand occurs long after the rulemaking docket has been closed and the staff has been reassigned. . . . The idea that an agency can or will quickly turn to remedying the factual or analytic defects in its remanded rule is surely naive, however minor those problems might appear in the abstract").

22. See, e.g., *Maine State Board of Education v. Cavazos,* 956 F.2d 376, 380, 382 (1st Cir. 1992); *Valley Citizens for a Safe Environment v. Aldridge,* 886 F.2d 458, 462–63 (1st Cir. 1989); but see Keith Schneider, "Courthouse Is a Citadel No Longer: U.S. Judges Curb Environmentalists," *N.Y. Times,* Mar. 23, 1992, at B7 (commenting on anti-regulatory attitude of conservative judges appointed to the federal bench in last decade).

23. See, e.g., *Chevron, Inc. v. Natural Resources Defense Council,* 467 U.S. 837, 844, 865 (1984) ("considerable weight should be accorded to an executive department's construction of a statutory scheme it is entrusted to administer"; "an agency to which Congress has delegated policymaking responsibilities may, within the limits of that delegation, properly rely upon the incumbent administration's views of wise policy to inform its judgments").

24. See RAND Corporation, *Trends in Tort Litigation Special Report* 25–29 (1987) (explaining that net compensation constitutes only about half of total expenditures for tort litigation); W. Kip Viscusi, "Toward a Diminished Role for Tort Liability: Social Insurance, Government Regulation, and Contemporary Risks to Health and Safety," 6 *Yale J. on Reg.* 65, 105–06 (1989) (criticizing tort system for lack of economies of scale and courts' lack of doctrines and expertise to assess properly probabilistic causation as factors making it inferior to regulation and social insurance as means for managing risks, especially in mass or toxic tort context); 28 U.S.C. §470 et seq. (mandating "Civil Justice Expense and Delay Reduction Plans").

25. See generally Jerry L. Mashaw, *Bureaucratic Justice* (1983). Mashaw concludes his analysis of agency workings with a vision of a "superbureau," which would employ elite public managers, oversee agency operations, and provide a model for bureaucratic governance. See id. at 226–27.
26. See 5 U.S.C. §3391 et seq.
27. Coherent control of the entire regulatory process would help ensure that the government would treat problems holistically and not, for example, clean up the ground by shifting pollution to the air. Cf. George C. Edwards III, *Implementing Public Policy* 134–41 (1980) (describing "fragmentation" of programs among numerous agencies and the tendency toward excessively narrow focus within each agency and toward inefficiency in the system and in achievement of program goals).
28. A Cross-Species Scaling Factor for Carcinogen Risk Assessment Based on Equivalence of mg/kg 3/4 /Day, 57 Fed. Reg. 24,152 (EPA, June 5, 1992) (draft report).
29. See Sheila Jasanoff, *The Fifth Branch: Science Advisers as Policymakers* 89–100 (1990) (discussing the role of the Science Advisory Board to the EPA in reviewing scientific evidence and recommending research strategies). See also Committee on the Institutional Means for Assessment of Risks to Public Health, National Research Council, *Risk Assessment in the Federal Government: Managing the Process*, 150–60 (1983) (recommending interagency coordination of cancer risk assessment broader than that EPA currently undertakes, but less comprehensive than that proposed here).
30. See Breyer, *Regulation and Its Reform*, at 36–59 (describing cost-of-service ratemaking and the choices regulators must make in determining rates); Thomas K. McCraw, *Prophets of Regulation* 239–270 (1984) (practice of cost-of-service ratemaking and its reform in electric power industry and airlines); see also Edwards, *Implementing Public Policy*, at 127–34 (describing "standard operating procedures" both as barriers to bureaucratic change and as aids in smooth adaptation to new policy challenges); see generally Alfred E. Kahn, *Economics of Regulation* (1988) (providing an economic and institutional analysis of traditional rate making issues).
31. Humphrey Taylor, "Confidence in Military Is Up While Confidence [in] the White House Falls," *The Harris Poll* (Mar. 22, 1992).
32. The FCCSET Ad Hoc Working Group on Risk Assessment, a high-level body set up in 1991, involving eleven federal agencies, is now in the process of attempting to pool experience and harmonize approaches. See EPA, *Intergovernmental Public Meeting on Risk Assessment in the Federal Government: Asking the Right Questions,* Final Report (June 10, 1992).
33. See Frank B. Cross, Daniel M. Byrd III, and Lester B. Lave, "Discernible Risk—A Proposed Standard for Significant Risk in Carcinogen Regulation," 43 *Admin. L. Rev.* 61 (1991) (discussing possible standards for identifying sig-

nificant risks); Federal Focus, Inc., *Toward Common Measures: Recommendations for a Presidential Executive Order in Environmental Risk Assessment and Risk Management Policy* 93–96 (1991); see generally Chris Whipple, ed., *De Minimis Risk* (1987).

34. EPA has set forth four different measures of "acceptable risk" in the proposal referred to: (1) a case-by-case approach based on a presumptive maximum individual risk of 1×10^{-4}; (2) a 1 case per year (across the entire U.S. population) maximum; (3) an invariable 1×10^{-4} maximum individual risk standard; and (4) a 1×10^{-6} maximum individual risk standard. EPA, National Emission Standards for Hazardous Air Pollutants, 53 Fed. Reg. 28,496, 28,523, 28,527, 28,529 (1988) (proposed rule and notice of public hearing); see also EPA, Airborne Radionuclides, 54 Fed. Reg. 9612 (1989) (same). Not surprisingly, courts have found such open-ended statutes to allow agencies substantial flexibility (and thus disparity) in determining permissible levels of substances posing health risks. *See American Textile Manufacturers' Inst. v. Donovan,* 452 U.S. 490, 508, 512 (1981) (OSHA provisions requiring standards to assure no "material impairment of health" to "the extent feasible" and "reasonably necessary or appropriate to provide safe or healthful employment" did not mandate cost-benefit analysis); cf. *Industrial Union Dep't, AFL-CIO v. American Petroleum Institute,* 448 U.S. 607, 642 (1980) (similar and noting that " 'safe' is not the equivalent of 'risk-free' "); see also *Hazardous Waste Treatment Council v. U.S. EPA,* 886 F.2d 355, 361–62 (D.C. Cir. 1989) (statute requiring EPA to make regulations to "minimize" threats to health did not require "levels at which it is conclusively presumed that no threat to health . . . exists" and permitted EPA to define " 'acceptable' level . . . 'below established levels of hazard' "); *Natural Resources Defense Council v. U.S. EPA,* 824 F.2d 1146, 1152–60 (D.C. Cir. 1987) (Congress's "ample margin of safety" requirement for EPA standard setting did not require a "zero level of emissions" standard or preclude consideration of "non-health-based considerations," including "cost and technological feasibility").

35. See also Committee on the Institutional Means for Assessment of Risks to Public Health, *Risk Assessment in the Federal Government,* at 162–75 (arguing for the development of "uniform inference guidelines" in cancer risk assessment, and for a central board on risk assessment to lead the process); Charles W. Powers, John A. Moore, and Arthur C. Upton, "Improving the Coherence of Federal Regulation of Risks from Hazardous Substances" 24–26 (1992) (revision of a draft paper originally prepared for the Carnegie Commission on Science, Technology, and Government) (discussing need for "inference guidelines").

36. See, e.g., Robert Cameron Mitchell and Richard T. Carson, "Valuing Drinking Water Risk Reductions Using the Contingent Valuation Method: A Methodological Study of Risks from THM and Giardia," (unpublished manuscript, 1986) (contingent valuation study with focus groups and in-depth interviews, using a

risk ladder—reproduced as Figure 1 in this book—as a visual aid). Mitchell and Carson found that a majority of respondents would vote against spending any extra money to reduce drinking water risks by 2.4 in 100,000. Id. at 66.

37. See Charles W. Powers, John A. Moore, and Arthur C. Upton, "Improving the Coherence of Federal Regulation of Risks from Hazardous Substances" 49–52 (1992) (revision of a draft paper originally prepared for the Carnegie Commission on Science, Technology and Government) (affirming need for a central organization to build a "Risk Inventory" of risk-related information). But cf. Carnegie Commission Staff Report, "Relative Risk and Regulation of Toxic Substances" 13–14 (Preliminary Draft, May 16, 1991), in *Task Force Binder* (May 24, 1991) (arguing for decentralized risk inventories located in various agencies). See also Sheila Jasanoff, *The Fifth Branch: Science Advisers as Policymakers* 85–122 (1990) (describing Science Advisory Board's emergence in the 1980s and cooperation with EPA as an independent source of scientific advice on, among other things, methodological issues).

38. See, e.g., John D. Graham, "Improving Chemical Risk Assessment," 14(4) *Regulation* 14, 15–16 (Fall 1991) (urging consideration of multiple factors in determining carcinogenic potency).

39. See, e.g., Adam M. Finkel, *Confronting Uncertainty in Risk Management: A Guide for Decision-Makers* (Resources for the Future, 1990); George M. Gray and John D. Graham, "Risk Assessment and Clean Air Policy," 10 *J. Policy Analysis & Mgmt.* 286 (1991) (suggesting use of range of estimates rather than simply upper-bound estimates); Adam M. Finkel, "Edifying Presentation of Risk Estimates: Not as Easy as It Seems," 10 *J. Policy Analysis & Mgmt.* 296 (1991); Dale Hattis and Robert L. Goble, "Expected Values for Projected Cancer Risks from Putative Genetically Acting Agents," 11 *Risk Analysis* 359 (1991) (discussing "upper confidence limits" and alternative models for communicating risk levels); Albert N. Nichols and Richard J. Zeckhauser, "The Perils of Prudence: How Conservative Risk Assessments Distort Regulation," *Regulation* 13, 21–24 (November/December 1986) (urging greater attention to the "expected value approach").

40. Recent scientific advances make this prospect increasingly likely. See, e.g., Gilbert S. Omenn, "Eco-Genetics: Genetics and Susceptibility to Cancer," 4(11) *Health & Environment Digest* 1 (January 1991); Gilbert S. Omenn, Curtis J. Omiecinski, and David L. Eaton, "Eco-Genetics of Chemical Carcinogens," in *Biotechnology and Human Genetic Predisposition to Disease* 81 (Charles R. Cantor et al., eds., 1991); A. G. Knudson, Jr., "Overview: Genes That Predispose to Cancer," 247 *Mutation Research* 185 (1991).

41. Such problems—and their possible solutions—also raise difficult ethical issues. See, e.g., Omenn, "Eco-Genetics," at 3 (citing sources).

42. See generally, Jasanoff, *The Fifth Branch,* ch. 5.

43. See, e.g., id., ch. 6; Committee on the Institutional Means for Assessment of Risks to Public Health, *Risk Assessment and the Federal Government,* at

144–48; Valerie M. Fogleman, "Regulating Science: An Evaluation of the Regulation of Biotechnology Research," 17 *Envtl. L.* 183, 250, 266 (1987) (describing EPA's successful use of independent advisory committees). There has also been some success with independent institutes such as the Health Effects Institute, funded by government and industry, which carries out research and literature reviews to produce reliable assessments of various regulatory strategies to aid governmental decision-making. See generally Charles W. Powers, "The Role of NGO's in Improving the Employment of Science and Technology in Environmental Management" (1991) (Working Paper, Carnegie Commission on Science, Technology, and Government). See also Charles W. Powers, "A History of the Health Effects Institute from the Viewpoint of an Interested Participant/Observer" (November 1991) (discussing history and activities of Health Effects Institute and Health Effects Institute—Asbestos Research).

44. See, e.g., U.S. Environmental Protection Agency, *Unfinished Business: A Comparative Assessment of Environmental Problems* (1987); Science Advisory Board, U.S. Environmental Protection Agency, *Reducing Risk: Setting Priorities and Strategies for Environmental Protection* (1990). See also Leslie Roberts, "Counting on Science at EPA," 249 *Science* 616 (1990) (discussing efforts to prioritize EPA programs); Richard L. Hembra, "Toxic Substances: EPA's Chemical Testing Program Has Not Resolved Safety Concerns," Statement before the Environment, Energy, and Natural Resources Subcommittee, Committee on Government Operations (March 18, 1992) (criticizing EPA's delay in implementing rationalizing procedures for regulatory decisions under the Federal Insecticide, Fungicide, and Rodenticide Act). But see Senator David Durenberger, "A Dissenting Voice," in *EPA Journal* (Mar./Apr. 1991) (criticizing EPA's conclusions in *Unfinished Business* and EPA SABs in *Reducing Risk*). EPA's Risk Assessment Council, based at EPA headquarters, "focuses on science policy issues that require coordination across EPA programs and may involve other regulatory agencies as well." Christopher J. Daggett, Robert E. Hazen, and Judith Auer Shaw, "Advancing Environmental Protection through Risk Assessment," 14 *Colum. J. Envtl. L.* 315, 317 (1989). EPA's guidelines harmonizing and publicizing the agency's exposure assessment methodology underwent review by its Risk Assessment Forum and Risk Assessment Council, external peer reviewers, the SAB, and the interagency Working Party on Exposure Assessment. EPA, Guidelines for Exposure Assessment, 57 Fed. Reg. 22,888 (May 29, 1992).

45. See 44 U.S.C. §3503 et seq. (establishing OIRA and defining some of its functions); Exec. Order No. 12,291, 3 C.F.R. §127 (1981) (mandating OMB cost-benefit analysis for major regulations); Exec. Order No. 12,498, 3 C.F.R. §327 (1986) (requiring agency to submit to OMB a "draft regulatory program," and applying this "early warning" requirement for "all significant regulatory actions" the agency plans for the year).

46. See Exec. Order No. 11,821, 3 C.F.R. §926 (1974) (requiring executive agencies to prepare inflation impact statements for regulations); Exec. Order No. 12,044, 3 C.F.R. §152 (1979) (requiring cost-benefit-based regulatory impact analysis). See also Harold H. Bruff, "Presidential Management of Agency Rulemaking," 57 *Geo. Wash. L. Rev.* 533, 546–49 (1989) (describing the Ford and Carter executive orders, and Carter's establishment of RARG, with CWPS support to oversee review under Exec. Order No. 12,044); Timothy B. Clark, "Carter's Assault on the Costs of Regulation," 10 *Nat'l J.* 1281 (1978) (Regulatory Analysis Review Group established to implement Exec. Order No. 12,044, chaired by chairman of the Council of Economic Advisers, includes heads of the principal economic and regulatory line agencies and OMB, but reviews regulations only after the agencies formally propose them); Timothy B. Clark, "How RARG has Regulated the Regulators," 11 *Nat'l J.* 1700 (1979) (describing the group's activities and assessing its impact on regulation); Carnegie Commission Staff Report, "Relative Risk and Regulation of Toxic Substances" 22–27 (preliminary draft, May 16, 1991), in *Task Force Binder* (May 24, 1991) (discussing coordinating organizations, such as OMB, RARG, Inter-Regulatory Liaison Group, Office of Science and Technology Policy); see generally Federal Focus, Inc., *Toward Common Measures: Recommendations for a Presidential Executive Order in Environmental Risk Assessment and Risk Management Policy* 28–48 (1991) (discussing White House efforts to coordinate risk assessment and risk management activities).

47. For this criticism see, e.g., David C. Vladeck, "O.M.B.: A Dangerous Super-agency," *N.Y. Times,* Sept. 6, 1989, at A25. For discussions of OIRA and its place in administrative law, see Harold H. Bruff, "Presidential Management of Agency Rulemaking," 57 *Geo. Wash. L. Rev.* 533, 549–95 (1989) (describing OMB and OMB-OIRA review in the Reagan era as generalist, budget-oriented, excessively secret, possibly biased toward industry, and a source of tension with agencies and Congress, but effective in subjecting regulation to presidential control and producing some promising institutional rearrangements and compromises offering better coordination and control of regulation); Christopher C. DeMuth and Douglas H. Ginsburg, "White House Review of Agency Rule-making," 99 *Harv. L. Rev.* 1075 (1986) (describing OMB review as an effective and efficient means for asking hard questions of agencies, setting priorities, and coordinating and assessing competing concerns in regulatory policy, while imposing little delay and blocking ill-advised regulations); Alan B. Morrison, "OMB Interference with Agency Rulemaking: The Wrong Way to Write a Regulation," 99 *Harv. L. Rev.* 1059 (1986) (criticizing OMB-OIRA review for delay, lack of substantive expertise, secrecy, and capture by regulated industries); Peter L. Strauss and Cass R. Sunstein, "The Role of the President and OMB in Informal Rulemaking," 38 *Admin. L. Rev.* 181 (1986) (arguing that OMB or something like it is needed as a method of presidential control over informal rule-making, bringing a broader perspective to bear on it and estab-

lishing coordination among efforts, but cautioning against intervention in the "general run of cases" and the risks of OMB's own unaccountability and political bias); see also Thomas O. McGarity, "Regulatory Analysis and Regulatory Reform," 65 *Tex. L. Rev.* 1243 (1987).

48. For a discussion about the desirability of placing coordinating authority in OMB or a related organization, see Charles W. Powers, John A. Moore, and Arthur C. Upton, "Improving the Coherence of Federal Regulation of Risks from Hazardous Substances" 53–56 (1992) (revision of a draft paper originally prepared for the Carnegie Commission on Science, Technology, and Government).

49. Council of Economic Advisors, *Economic Report of the President 1990* 193–97 (GPO, 1990). In 1992, another Presidential council, the Council on Competitiveness, has also been active in this area, although with limited effect. See Keith Schneider, "White House Drops Plan on Setting Health Risks," *N.Y. Times,* July 28, 1992, at A9 (describing the Council's abortive proposal for a new scientific oversight group and new assumptions in risk assessment); "Mr. Quayle's Irregular Regulation," *N.Y. Times,* Dec. 15, 1991, at D14 (discussing environmentalist concerns about secrecy and deregulatory bias in the Council).

50. The FCCSET Ad Hoc Working Group on Risk Assessment has a broad mission to harmonize approaches and reduce uncertainty in risk assessment by improving scientific methods, but is not concerned with the policy questions of risk management. See DHHS and EPA, Risk Assessment Practices in the Federal Government, 56 Fed. Reg. 54580-82 (Oct. 22, 1991) (establishing it), and EPA, *Asking the Right Questions* (summarizing its progress and ongoing work after nine months). For examples of interagency task forces with narrower mandates, see National Toxicology Program, Draft Response of the Program to Recommendations in the Final Report of the Advisory Review by the NTP Board of Scientific Counselors, 57 Fed. Reg. 61,439 (Dec. 24, 1992) (ongoing review by scientific oversight body, assisted by ad hoc expert consultants, of selection and prioritization of chemicals for testing, and of testing methods); EPA, Visibility Impairment from Pollution: Public Meetings of Interagency Task Force on Visibility, 49 Fed. Reg. 44,770 (Nov. 9, 1984); EPA and Department of the Army, Memorandum of Agreement, 55 Fed. Reg. 5510 (Feb. 15, 1990); EPA, Interagency Policy on the Beneficial Use of Municipal Sewage Sludge on Federal Land, 56 Fed. Reg. 33186, 33186 (July 10, 1991) (announcing the uniform policy and scientific understandings of seven agencies and departments, developed by an interagency task force that was convened by OMB in 1990, on the beneficial use of municipal sewage sludge).

51. See generally M. Gerteis and S. Thomas, "The Interagency Regulatory Liaison Group," in Landy, Roberts, and Thomas, eds., *E.P.A.: Asking the Wrong Questions?* (1990). For a brief discussion of the group's efforts to harmonize cancer risk evaluation across agencies, see Committee on Institutional Means for Assessments of Risks to Public Health, National Research Council, *Risk Assessment in the Federal Government,* at 60–62. For examples of its output,

see Interagency Agreement, 42 Fed. Reg. 54,856 (1977) (agreement to coop-
erate on regulation of toxic substances); Interagency Work Plan, 43 Fed. Reg.
7174–78 (1978) (on risk assessment). For contemporary descriptions, see, e.g.,
"Regulation: Carter Starts to Turn a Supertanker," *The Economist,* Apr. 14,
1979, at 42; Ernest Holsendolph, "The U.S. Drive—Deregulation," *N.Y. Times,*
Oct. 7, 1980, at D1.

52. See Paul M. Falcone, *Familiarisation with the French Administration* (1987)
(describing Conseil structure, practices, procedures, and recruitment channels,
and attributing Conseil's prestige and authority to elite composition, members'
mix of experience and expertise, and its combination of judicial and consultative roles); Bureau d'Information du Public, *The Conseil d'Etat, Structure
and Role* (1984) (describing formal structure and career path of the Conseil);
L. Neville Brown and J. F. Garner, *French Administrative Law* (1983)
(describing the Conseil, with an emphasis on its judicial functions); but see
Christopher Edley, Jr., *Administrative Law: Rethinking Judicial Control of
Bureaucracy* (1990) 241–45 (noting that the Conseil, in its judicial capacity,
operates without the checks formal separation of powers imposes on U.S.
courts, and that Conseil members enjoy great, if informal, security of tenure,
but finding "the same [theme] of deference to [agency] expertise . . . so promi-
nent in United States law," and not the "strikingly different jurisprudence" the
author expected); Stephen F. Williams, "The Roots of Deference," 100 *Yale
L.J.* 1103, 1105 (1991) (reviewing Christopher Edley, Jr., *Administrative Law:
Rethinking Judicial Control of Bureaucracy* (1990), attributing the similar levels of deference to expertise in the Conseil and U.S. courts to the "disadvan-
tage" a "generalist, multimembered, and reactive" body is at when it confronts
an agency "specialist on the latter's turf").

53. Herbert Kaufman, *The Forest Ranger: A Study in Administrative Behavior*
155–56, 176–83 (1960).

54. Some of the foundations for such a structure are already in place. First, a number
of science-related posts in government have already come to be recognized as
especially vital, prestigious, demanding of scientific expertise and political
acumen, and requiring close and often informal coordination across departmen-
tal and branch lines. See John H. Trattner, *The Prune Book: The 60 Toughest
Science and Technology Jobs in Washington* (1992) (describing science-related
jobs in the executive office of the president, executive departments and agencies,
and in Congress, formal and informal duties and important formal and informal
relationships with other arms of government, the scientific community, and the
public). Second, the Executive Branch already recognizes some of the values
of rotation, although for too few administrators, at too advanced a stage in their
careers, and among those with waning policy influence in the Senior Executive
Service. See Joel D. Aberbach and Bert A. Rockman, "What Has Happened to
the U.S. Senior Civil Service?" *Brookings Rev.* 35 (Fall 1990) (describing
the Civil Service Reform Act of 1978's creation of greater flexibility in moving

SES executive among posts, but also describing the continuing decline, since the early 1970s, in senior civil servants' sense that they influence policy and attributing that decline to growing financial constraints on government and the problems of divided government); see also Frances H. Irwin, "An Integrated Framework for Preventing Pollution and Protecting the Environment," 22 *Envtl. L.* 1, 65 (1991) ("changing criteria for advancement of managers in the Senior Executive Service to credit experience in different types of programs, on Agency-wide task forces, and in different locations clearly has made EPA a different place from that described in a 1984 report: 'Many EPA employees are currently prisoners to their career specialties and their geographic locations'") (citations omitted).

55. Thomas Jefferson, *Letter to William Charles Jarvis,* in John Bartlett, *Familiar Quotations* 473 (14th ed. 1968); see also Clayton P. Gillette and James E. Krier, "Risk, Courts, and Agencies," 138 *U. Penn. L. Rev.* 1027, 1101–04 (1990) (describing expanded roles for a technocratic elite of agency experts in managing increasingly complex and scientific-technological risks as a threat to democracy, and suggesting greater public participation in risk management as a possible solution).

56. Jean-Jacques Rousseau, *The Social Contract,* Book II, ch. 7; cf. id., Book III, ch. 4.

57. See Jerry L. Mashaw, "Prodelegation: Why Administrators Should Make Political Decisions," 1 *J. Law, Econ. & Org.* 81, 95–98 (1985) (arguing that broad delegation of regulatory authority from Congress to Executive is compatible with democratic legitimacy and greater accountability because it leads to rules less vague than statutes typically are, and rules for which the President may be held electorally accountable). Compare Bronwen Maddox, "The Cost of Fear," *Financial Times,* Oct. 7, 1992, at 10 ("The choice of the tolerable level of risk is a matter for voters and politicians. But in putting figures on the reasons for fear, from a position beyond the heat of environmental debate, the formal assessment of risk does at least start to make the choices intelligible").

58. This assumption may be optimistic, for real pay in the civil service has tended to decline—see National Commission on the Public Service (Paul A. Volcker, Chairman), *Leadership for America: Rebuilding the Public Service* 35 (Congressional Committee Reprint 101-4, Committee on Post Office and Civil Service, H.R., May 2, 1989) ("Between 1969 . . . and 1988, the purchasing power of executive, judicial, and legislative salaries fell by 35 percent")—and working conditions include "ethics" rules that may be unreasonably restrictive. See, e.g., Office of Government Ethics, "Standards of Ethical Conduct for Employees of the Executive Branch," 56 Fed. Reg. 33,778, 33,809 (July 2, 1991) (proposed rule, to be codified at 5 CFR §2635.704) (expansive definition of Government property, including office supplies, telephone communications, and library materials, which may be used only for a very narrow range of

authorized purposes); *Stanek v. Department of Transportation,* 805 F.2d 1572 (Fed. Cir. 1986) (upholding dismissal of employee for, inter alia, using government word-processing equipment to write three pages of personal correspondence and fifty-nine pages related to "whistleblowing" activities); P. Broida, *A Guide to Merit Systems Protection Board Law and Practice* 797–800 (1990) (collecting cases of draconian punishment for small-scale abuses of government property). Cf. Volcker Commission, *supra,* at 14, 15 ("Codes of conduct . . . should be simple and straightforward"; "the financial disclosure process, while a key protection against conflicts of interest, should be streamlined to ease the burdens on potential appointees").

59. See Peter Passell, "Experts Question Staggering Costs of Toxic Cleanups," *N.Y. Times,* Sept. 1, 1991, at A1, A28 (discussing proposal of Dan Dudek, an economist with the Environmental Defense Fund, that, instead of communities being taxed to pay for extra cleanup effort, affected communities be offered a portion, perhaps 20 percent, of the savings associated with less-than-total repair; the communities could then choose to spend this money to save lives in other ways).

60. Cf. Lester B. Lave, "Does the Surgeon General Need a Statistics Advisor?" in 3 *Chance: New Directions for Statistics and Computing* 33, 35 (1990) (noting that political policy maker has a time horizon of three months, but that effective risk regulation requires longer time horizon).

61. See Arthur S. Miller, "Pretense and Our Two Constitutions," 54 *Geo. Wash. L. Rev.* 375, 381–82 (1986) (defining "iron triangle" as "issue networks" that "provide the means by which public policy is made" and "consist[ing] of the industry or other group being regulated or affected by legislation, the relevant administrative agency and the congressional committee[s] having jurisdiction over the agency [and thus the industry]"); see generally Gordon Adams, *The Politics of Defense Contracting: The Iron Triangle* (1981).

62. See Breyer and Stewart, *Administrative Law and Regulatory Policy,* ch. 8 (2d ed., 1985).

63. Franklin D. Roosevelt, *Address at Oglethorp University,* in John Bartlett, *Familiar Quotations* 970 (14th ed., 1968).

64. See Stephen Breyer, "Judicial Review of Questions of Law and Policy," 38 *Ad. L. Rev.* 363, 394–97 (1986).

65. See generally Stephen Breyer, "On the Uses of Legislative History in Interpreting Statutes," 65 *S. Cal. L. Rev.* 845 (1992).

INDEX